W9-BJB-639

CORY EVERSON'S WORKOUT

Most Perigee Books are available at special quantity discounts for bulk purchases for sales promotions, premiums, fund-raising or educational use. Special books, or book excerpts, can also be created to fit specific needs.

For details, write: Special Markets: The Berkley Publishing Group, 375 Hudson Street, New York, New York 10014.

CORY EVERSON'S WORKOUT

Corinna Everson
with Jeff Everson, Ph.D.

Photography by Ralph DeHaan

A Perigee Book

WARNING!
The exercises in this book are intended only for
healthy people. People with health problems should
not follow these routines without a physician's
approval. Before beginning any exercises or dietary
program, always consult with your doctor.

A Perigee Book
Published by The Berkley Publishing Group
A division of Penguin Putnam Inc.
375 Hudson Street
New York, NY 10014

A Wellington Press Book

Copyright © 1991 by Corinna Everson and Jeff Everson, Ph.D.
Cover design by Mike Stromberg

All rights reserved. This book, or parts thereof,
may not be reproduced in any form without permission.
Published simultaneously in Canada

First edition: October 1991

The Penguin Putnam Inc. World Wide Web site address is
http://www.penguinputnam.com

Library of Congress Cataloging-in-Publication Data

Everson, Corinna.
    [Workout]
    Cory Everson's workout / Corinna Everson with Jeff Everson.
        p.   cm.
    "A Perigee book."
    Includes index.
    ISBN: 0-399-51684-0 (alk. paper)
        1. Weight training. 2. Physical fitness. 3. Bodybuilding.
    I. Everson, Jeff.   II. Title
    GV546.E94   1991   91-15310 CIP
    613.7'13 — dc20

Printed in the United States of America
   14   15   16   17   18   19   20

This book is printed on acid-free paper.
            ∞

Acknowledgments

To Jeff. He's the reason I have this book. Jeff is part of everything I am and do.
To our families whom we love as they love us.

To super-agents Scott Dmitrenko and Brian Zevnik.
To photographer Ralph DeHaan.

To my personal assistant, Laura "Lester" Gorman.
To Darci Dmitrenko, training partner, friend and doodle.
To Warner Center Athletic Club.

To Billie Boy, Bolaro, Shilo, White Guy, Ricky, Dr. Beaver, Wolf, Koala, Ingenué and Heady.

To all my wonderful fans who have blessed me with their love and support.

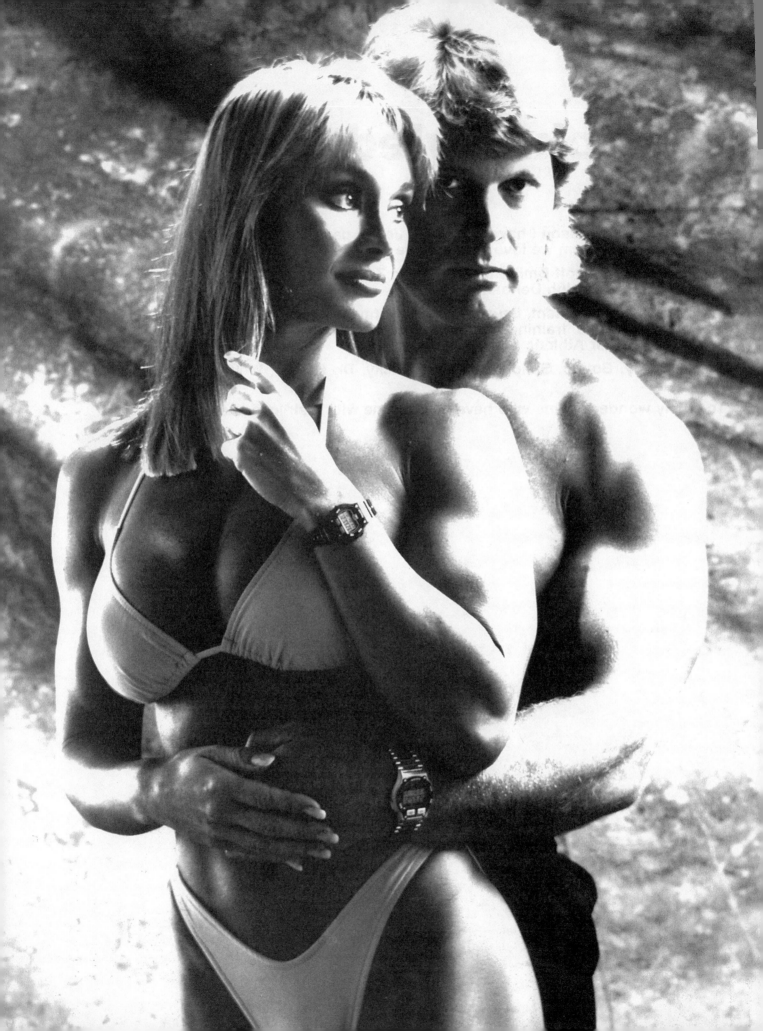

Contents

While Cory poses, her husband, Jeff, seems intent
on practicing the Heimlich maneuver!

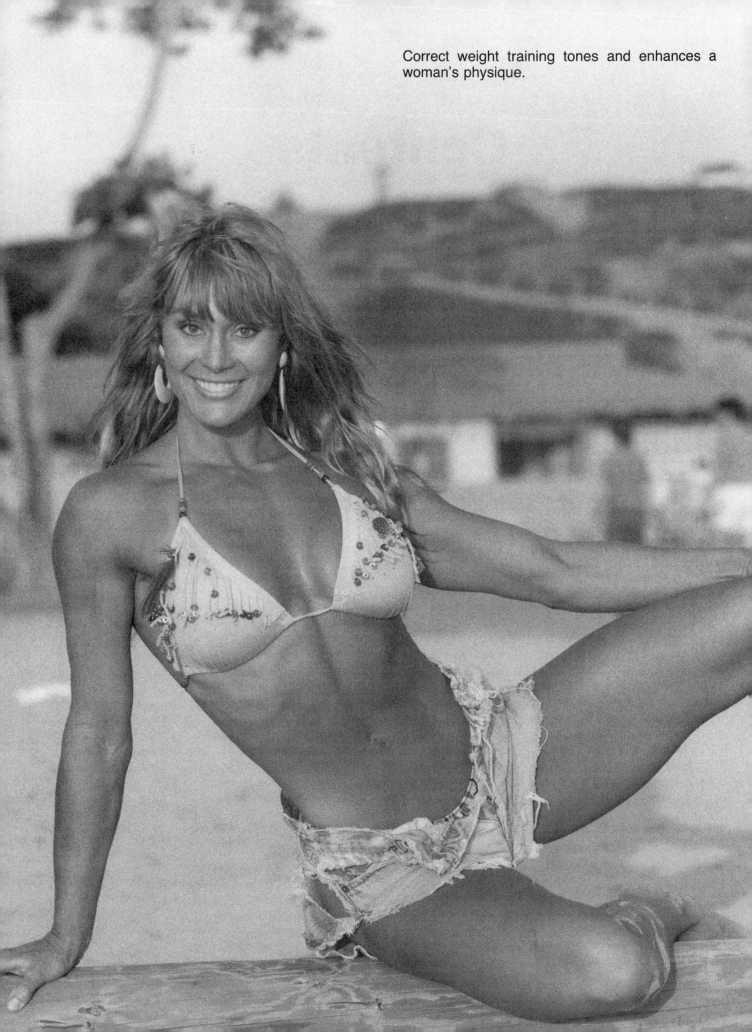

Correct weight training tones and enhances a woman's physique.

1

WHAT TO EXPECT

Despite many articles in magazines, newspapers and books on exercise and fitness, most of you have a lot of trouble putting together your workout plan. You don't know how to work out or what to expect from your training. You know that walking, jogging and cutting back on fat and cholesterol are all important. However, when it comes to customizing a workout for your goals and lifestyle, or starting weight training, most of you are lost sheep.

BASIC ISSUES

I've been involved in fitness for 12 years and wherever I go, I hear the same questions: If I lift weights, will I lose my femininity? Will I get big muscles? Can I eat bread and red meat? How many days should I work out? How many exercises should I do? How many sets and repetitions should I do? How much weight should I use? How long should I work out? I'm pregnant; will I hurt my baby? Can I get strong without adding bulk? Should I do aerobics before or after weight training? Does cross training work?

Your biggest concerns always seem to be about losing femininity (except you guys reading this), toning without gaining bulk and losing fat in your "problem" body areas (hips, rear, thighs and waist). I think you have to be comfortable with these basic issues before we deal with the amount of weight you should use, how many days you should train, the number of sets and repetitions you should do and what a good diet is.

FEMININITY AND BEAUTY

The lines "Beauty is in the eye of the beholder" and "A thing of beauty is a joy forever" are self-evident. Being born a woman means you are feminine. Exercise, good health and fitness can't change gender. There is no better definition of a beautiful body than an efficient body.

Your heart is beautiful when it's healthy and works. Your body is beautiful when it's in shape, without unhealthy fat. Muscles are beautiful because they perform. Beauty is everything working! An old Chevy that runs is more beautiful than a $220,000 Rolls Royce that doesn't run, especially if you're in the middle of nowhere.

Weight training is the best way to beautify your body. It creates sexy contours, making you leaner and less fat. With circuit weight training, you get fit inside and out.

Real beauty isn't cosmetic. It's not fat suctioning, silicone implants or designer clothes. These might make you look beautiful, but they aren't real, are they? With those things, you hide your real self. Fitness is real beauty! With exercise and fitness, you don't hide, you reveal yourself.

Definitions and standards change. The

beautiful women of the Renaissance period would be considered obese today! Shamefully, today's fitness paragons are toothpick-thin models. In a Renaissance reversal, many of these skinflints eat poorly and use diuretics and laxatives to keep their weight down.

HULK HOGAN

Some of you are actually afraid of exercise. You believe that weight training will blow your muscles up like those of professional wrestler Hulk Hogan. Many of you think muscle destroys femininity and beauty, yet women are born with just as many muscles as men.

It's not easy for women to get larger muscles from exercise. You will get stronger, more flexible, toned and have a better shape. You will lose fat but you won't always get bigger muscles!

It's extremely difficult for an average woman to develop muscles like a competitive bodybuilder. I competed in sports for many years and was a bodybuilder for five years before I won my first of six Ms. Olympia titles. Professional bodybuilders are the cream of the crop in building muscles. In fact, even when I reached that level, my muscle size and definition was only average compared to some of my competitors!

WHAT ABOUT COMPETITIVE BODYBUILDING?

When I was competing from 1979 to 1989, I read a few articles that said women's muscles were unfeminine, ugly and unhealthy. Everyone is entitled to their opinion, but is muscle development uglier and less healthy than unsightly mounds of blubber or skin and bones and no energy? Is athletic ability less feminine than weakness, frailty and poor coordination?

When I was bodybuilding, no one ever told me I was unfeminine. Instead, some people told me I didn't look like "those lady bodybuilders in the magazines"; yet I was the number-one lady in bodybuilding! A radio announcer once asked me, "If women lift heavy weights, will they grow a moustache?" I said, "No, we grow tails and

pin them on donkeys like you."

I've been an athlete all my life and never worried about femininity. Do you think tennis star Jennifer Capriatti worries that her forearms are masculine because she serves four times faster than the average man? Did Mary Lou Retton lose her femininity when she vaulted her way to Olympic gold in gymnastics in 1984?

Unfortunately, when someone writes a bigoted story about fit women, or when fitness magazines only show pictures of women bodybuilders the day of the contest, after they have dieted into a super-defined condition, you don't get the true picture.

Don't get the idea that you will automatically end up looking like competitive bodybuilders if you train with weights. That requires extraordinary dedication and effort. You will get leaner, with improved shape and better proportion, from weight training. Although I now have more muscle and less fat than when I was in high school, my weight is the same as it was when I graduated!

WHERE IS COMPETITIVE BODYBUILDING HEADING?

Competitive bodybuilding gets a bum rap, but at times, I'm embarrassed by the sport. Our magazines don't do female bodybuilders any favors with the general public when they photograph bodybuilders when their body fat is so low. Physique contests don't measure our athletic ability, talent or coordination. There's little agreement on scoring posing, which frustrates competitors and fans.

Steroid use is another black eye. With my sports cross-training background, it's hard to understand how women build more muscle than I had in heavy training, but, many did (and do). In some cases, women have been accused of "looking just like men," and have gone too far, unnaturally. It's not their muscle size or definition so much as it is their voices. Some women make James Earl Jones sound like a tenor. By their own admission, some women have used bushelsful of anabolic steroids, dangerous hormone drugs that make you build much larger muscles faster.

Steroids could destroy men's and wom-

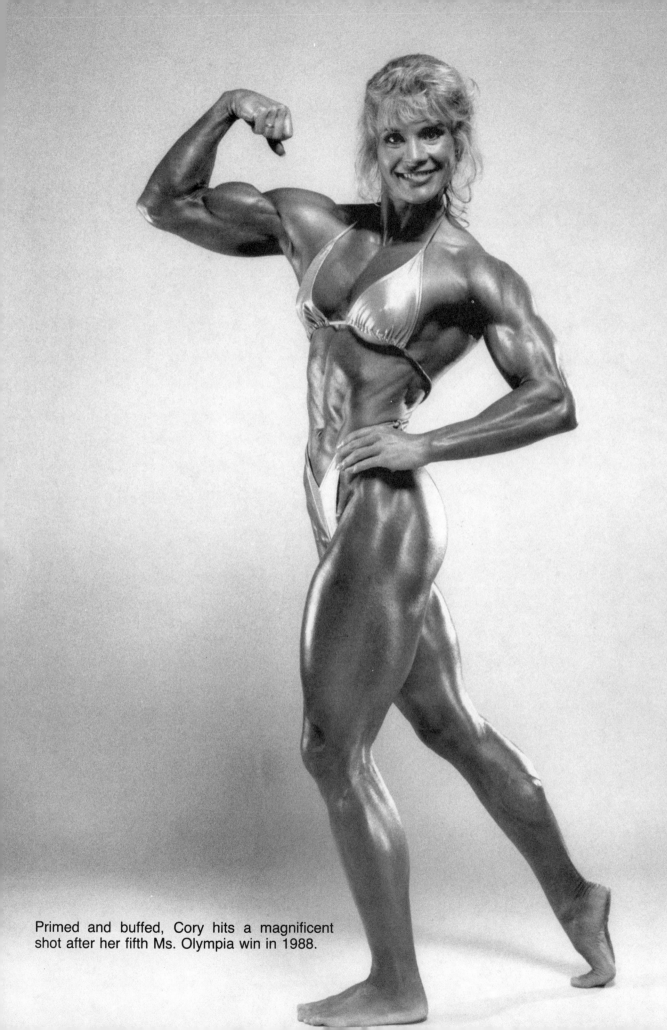

Primed and buffed, Cory hits a magnificent shot after her fifth Ms. Olympia win in 1988.

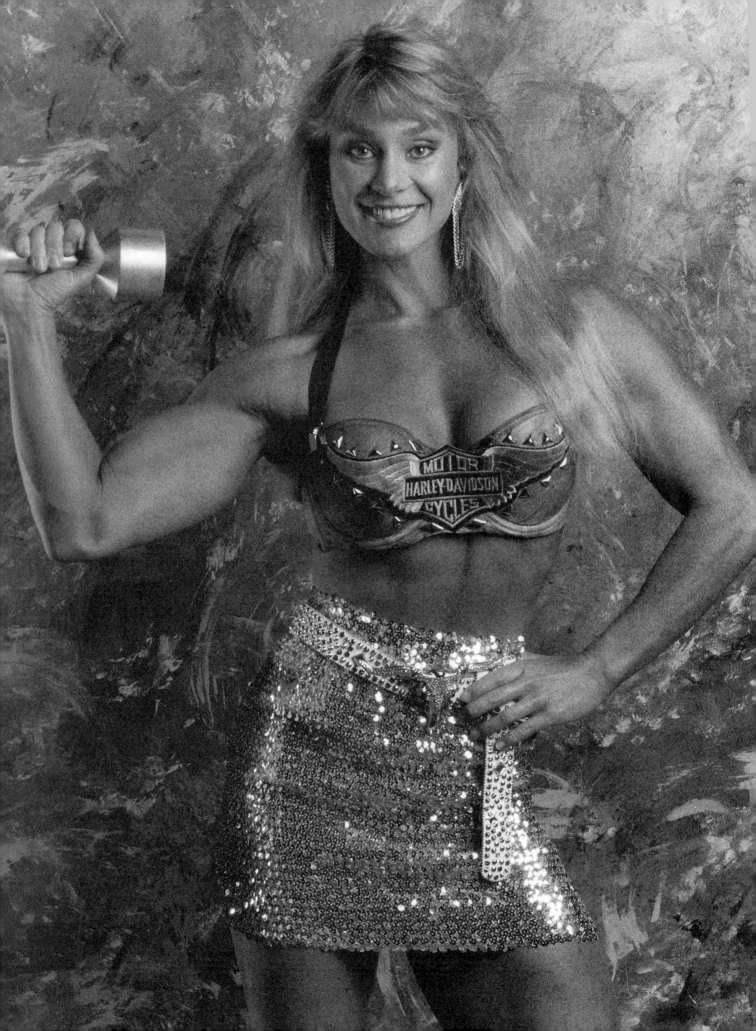

en's bodybuilding. They have *no* justifiable role in sports—for any purpose.

ALICE IN WONDERLAND

Erroneous fitness statements by educated people make me cringe. Two researchers from San Diego State University wrote in *US News & World Report:* "Bodybuilding without doing aerobics and stretching is not a good idea. It [bodybuilding] produces large but tight and injury-prone muscles that also lack endurance."

Nonsense! Even if bodybuilding did what they say, it would still be much better than no exercise. Still, they are as wrong as rain. Bodybuilding does *not* produce tight muscles. I'm just as flexible now as I was when competing in gymnastics years ago. Bodybuilding increases your flexibility and most women can't get big muscles (most men can't either).

Common sense should tell people that weak, unconditioned muscles are the ones that are injury-prone, not strong, flexible muscles! Bodybuilders have tremendous muscle endurance. Who would last longer carrying 100-pound blocks all day long, a bodybuilder or a marathon runner? Each time the runner carries one, it takes so much effort that he fatigues quickly and can't recover (if he's able to carry one at all)! The conditioned bodybuilder carries more blocks for a longer time (more endurance) because the weight of the block is relatively much less to him. With a 10-pound block, the marathoner lasts longer. Obviously, endurance is relative.

A medical doctor quoted in a large newspaper wrote: "I recommend machines rather than dumbbells and free bars used by bodybuilders. An exercise-based machine program can be set up by a trained instructor at a reputable gym. If followed conscientiously, it will provide conditioning without creating the large and bulky—*hence, not very useful muscles* [emphasis mine] normally associated with bodybuilding."

More nonsense. What does "not very useful muscles" mean? If you have an av-

erage IQ of 100, does that mean someone with a 140 IQ has "not very useful brain cells" just because he has more or can better use the ones he has? Fortunately, most doctors aren't stupid about exercise and weight training. There's evidence that the bigger your muscles, the better!

In The Health Letter Lawrence Lamb, M.D., writes: "Muscle is critical to your health and energy level. Think of muscle cells as energy cells of your body. Individuals with poor muscle development, such as the out-of-shape office worker, have low energy levels. Lack of muscle makes it easier to gain fat, despite calorie restriction below levels for proper nutrition. Adequate muscle helps posture and appearance. Loss of muscle is associated with aging, while good musculature is associated with vibrant youth."

Dr. Lamb notes that at rest, fat does not use as many calories as muscle tissue. Often, people become fat with age not because of what they eat, how much they eat, or their inactivity, but because they use less calories at rest than they used to use when they had more muscle! Since you have less muscle with age, you become like the character in *Alice in Wonderland* who had to run just to stay in the same place!

Use weights, keep your muscle and burn more calories maintaining that muscle! So much for the "not very useful muscles" of bodybuilders. In fact, the bigger your muscles, the more calories they burn and the harder it is for you to get fat! Less fat means better health.

Follow some of the personalized workouts in this book and you'll quickly find beauty, fitness and health.

SEE YOUR DOCTOR FIRST!

See your doctor if you are starting any fitness program (especially if you are over 35 and inactive). Do this for advice with your program if you have any special conditions requiring medical guidance.

Your doctor will measure your blood pressure; listen to your lungs for breathing problems and your heart for irregularities such as strange heart sounds, valve problems or abnormal beats; check for blood problems, neuromuscular or musculo-

Cory primes her biceps so she can control her Harley on the highway.

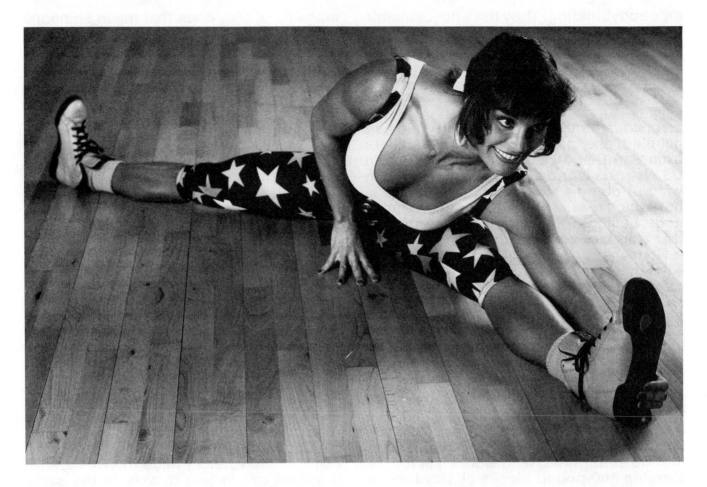

If you're not Gumby, this might be kind of hard. This is an advanced stretch for your hamstrings and inner-thigh muscles.

skeletal problems and metabolic diseases like diabetes or other blood sugar conditions.

A blood sample will give him information about your kidneys, liver, cholesterol, triglycerides and red and white blood-cell levels. He will ask for a health history which will help establish the safety of your exercise program.

Don't skip your physical!

WHAT EXERCISE CAN DO: THE FACTS!

- Between 1.5 and 2 million people in the USA will have heart attacks this year; 500,000–700,000 people will die, over 300,000 before they even get to the hospital. Many of these people suffer from high blood pressure and don't even know it.
- **Heart disease causes almost half the deaths in the USA in any one year!**
- **Almost 50 percent of these heart attacks are in people under 65.**
- **Strokes kill over 160,000 people each year.**
- **Cancer is the second biggest killer, but is gaining rapidly on heart disease in all age groups.**
- **Nutrition affects heart disease, strokes and some forms of cancer.**

It might surprise you that exercise has a direct effect on these diseases. Exercise increases your muscle strength, endurance, power, flexibility, shape, tone, posture and proportion. Exercise rehabilitates and prevents injuries and slows aging. Exercise keeps your metabolic rate up by maintaining muscle and thins your blood, lowers your blood cholesterol (particularly your bad cholesterol), and helps sugar metabolism and blood pressure. Exercise reduces anxiety, tension and anger reactions to stress.

Weight workouts help older individuals

too! They build strength and endurance, helping their agility and self-reliance. Weight training helps bone thickness, strength and health. Supervised workouts can help diabetes, heart disease, arthritis, multiple sclerosis and other muscle-wasting diseases. Exercise pumps blood and oxygen through your joints and muscles and increases your circulation.

Exercise improves your body composition. Obesity is related to some cancers, heart disease, stroke, diabetes and other diseases. Since exercise controls obesity, it fights these diseases.

Exercise, with special breathing techniques, increases your lung power. Working out increases your abdominal, intercostal and trapezius muscle control, assisting breathing. Spinal-cord patients improve their breathing with weight workouts.

At one time or another, most people suffer back pain or disability. Weight training (and aerobics) reduces back pain or prevents it in almost all cases.

Recovering from surgery and childbirth is quicker and easier when you're fit. Physically active people suffer less colon, breast and reproductive cancers (this also may be associated with the low-fat diets that fitness-minded individuals follow). Exercise cannot cure cancer, but it may help the quality of life during the disease.

Don't be afraid to exercise, it will only do you good. So stay tuned, my workouts have double benefits—inside and out.

As sturdy as her Mexican-style Bell Canyon, California, home, Cory flexes a powerful bicep on a warm summer day.

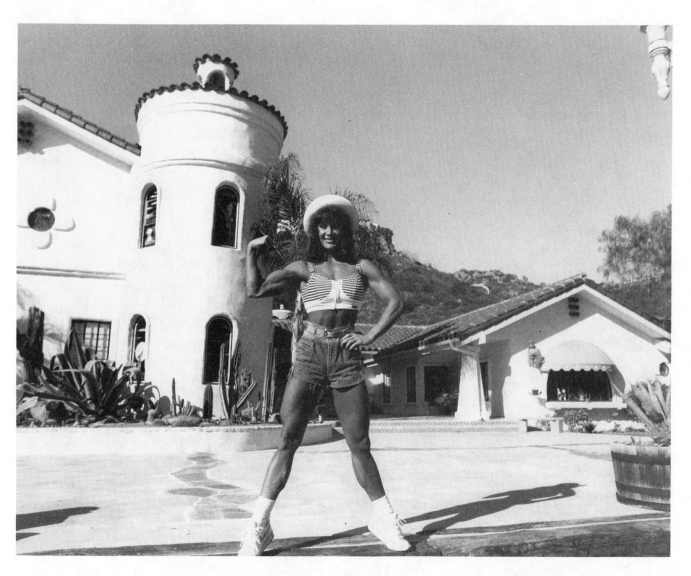

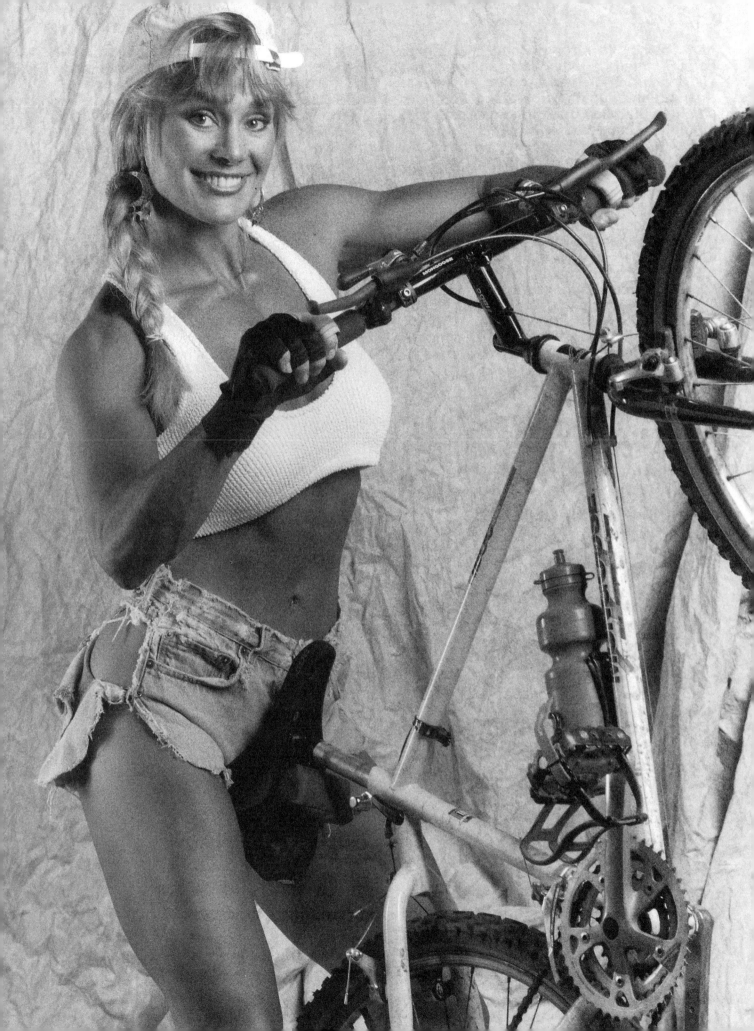

2
A MOUSE IN A MAZE?

My goal is to make exercise less confusing. Exercise and fitness workouts must be fun and have purpose or they're too boring. Don't start my workouts like a mouse in a maze. Don't be mixed up over terms. Refer to my definitions. They'll help you understand fitness terms that you don't recognize (and there will be plenty). I recommend that you read this chapter very carefully—with your thinking cap on!

Abds: Short for abdominal muscles. Your "abds" rotate and flex your upper body forward and sideways, and assist breathing and upper-body stability. Your abdominals are comprised of your rectus abdominis, internal and external obliques and transversus abdominis.
Abduction: Sideways movement of your arm or leg away from your body.
Adduction: Movement of your arm or leg back toward the center of your body.
Adipose Tissue: A fancy name for fat!
Advanced Workout: Workouts for someone who has been working out correctly for at least one year.
Aerobic: Endurance exercise where oxygen is used to produce energy. Nonstop exercise for at least 20 minutes to elevate your heart rate to 60–80 percent of your maximum. An example is cross-country skiing.

Agility: A measure of fitness. The ability to change directions and speed of movement quickly. Coordination.
Amino Acids: The constituents of proteins. The essential amino acids must be provided by your diet. Nonessential amino acids can be made by your body.

Chicken breasts are high in protein, low in fat and relatively low in calories.

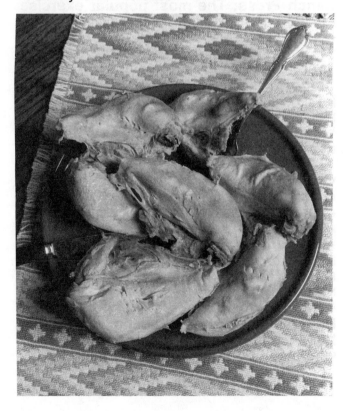

Cory looking toned doing a "wheelie" with her mountain bike.

Anabolic: Building or promoting growth.

Anabolic Steroid: A drug that increases protein formation for muscle strength and size (when combined with exercise and adequate calories).

Anaerobic: Short-burst exercise with non-oxygen energy sources. Exercise that does not significantly elevate your heart rate for long periods of time. An example is powerlifting.

Androgens: Steroid sex hormones promoting male sexual characteristics.

Antagonist: The muscle that relaxes when the opposite muscle (called the agonist) produces movement. Your triceps relaxes while your biceps contracts to produce forearm flexion.

ATP: A chemical that provides energy for muscle contraction. It must be manufactured and can't be stored in your body.

Atrophy: A decrease in muscle size.

Balance: The ability to keep your body steady. In physique parlance, harmony of all your muscle groups.

Barbell: The shaft connecting weight plates and collars. A regular bar with collars weighs about 20 pounds. The bigger Olympic bar with collars weighs 55 pounds!

Beginner Workout: Workouts designed for someone with less than six months of correct, regular workouts.

Bench Press: The most popular exercise for your chest muscles.

Biceps: The muscle in your upper arm that flexes and supinates your forearm (turns your palm up).

Blood Pressure: A ratio of pressures, known as systolic pressure to diastolic pressure. Systolic is the pressure of your blood against your artery walls when your heart contracts. Average values are 105–130 millimeters of mercury. Diastolic is the vessel pressure when your heart is relaxed or filling. Average values are 75–85 millimeters of mercury. High blood pressure is also called hypertension. Essential hypertension is high blood pressure with no known cause.

BMR: Your basal metabolic rate is the number of calories you use in a twenty-four-hour rest period.

Bodybuilding: Weight training workouts to build muscle. Also, organized competition where competitors pose and are judged on physiques.

Body-Fat Percentage: Your body fat, as opposed to muscle, connective tissue or bone. For males, 20–35 percent is average (although too high). For women, 25–45 percent is average (also too high).

Brachialis: The powerhouse flexor of your forearm. It is strongest when your forearm is lifted up with your hand in mid-position.

Brown Fat: Theoretically, a type of body fat that contributes energy calories more efficiently than regular fat.

Calorie: The unit of heat expanded in energy metabolism. Food is measured in calories by its ability to provide this heat. There are about 90 calories in an average apple.

Calves: The muscle groups in the back of your lower legs.

Carb Loading: Eating to super-compensate your body with stored carbohydrates for increased energy production.

Carbohydrates: One of three main food nutrients your body needs for energy, growth and maintenance. "Carbs" are combinations of sugars and starches.

Cardiovascular Workout: Workouts stressing your heart, lungs and coronary circulation. Synonymous with aerobic exercise.

Cholesterol: A waxy substance produced by your body and also obtained through food. Too much cholesterol in your blood may predispose you to a heart attack!

Circuit Workout: A series of different exercises with little or no rest.

Clavicle: Your collarbone.

Concentric Contraction: Another name for muscle shortening. Also called positive exercise. When your muscle lengthens against resistance, it's contracting eccentrically.

Contraction: A muscle contraction where the muscle fibers shorten, produce force and move bones; or where muscles lengthen against resistance (also called negative or eccentric exercise); or where muscle force is exerted against a fixed object. In the latter case, there's no movement but there is an isometric contraction.

Cool-Down Period: Very light movement and stretching following your exercise which brings your heart rate to normal and prevents blood from pooling in your legs

Always wear a belt when you train heavy—not over the shoulder, but around your waist!

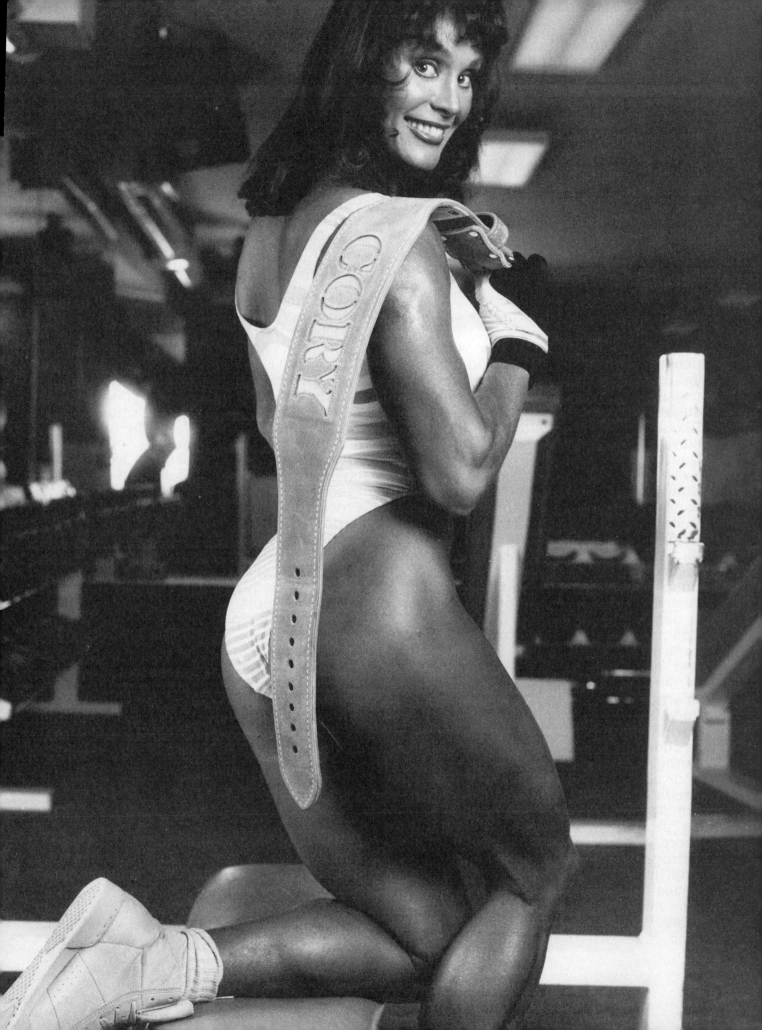

which might cause dizziness and blackout.

Cross Training: Aerobic exercise when your sport is primarily anaerobic, and vice versa. Also, a variety of workouts to improve performance and fitness.

Cutting Up: Slang for defining and losing body fat, but trying to keep your muscle at the same time.

Cycle Workouts: Rotating workouts to stress intensity or volume and, at other times, toning.

Deads: Short for deadlifts, lifts for your lower back, glutes and leg muscles.

Definition: Muscle without visible fat.

Delts: Short for deltoids, your shoulder muscles. Delts are divided into your front, middle and rear heads.

Density: The hardness and thickness of your muscles.

Diabetes: A medical condition where your pancreas does not produce enough insulin. Exercise can help many diabetics because exercise burns up excess blood sugar.

Diastolic Blood Pressure: See Blood Pressure.

Double-Split Workout: Working out twice a day, but training different body parts.

Dumbbell: The small minibar used in each hand in weight workouts.

Duration: The length of your workout.

Ectomorph: An individual who is naturally thin with little muscle and a light bone frame.

Endomorph: An individual who has a heavy bone frame and a greater tendency to add body fat.

Endurance: The ability to carry on muscle contractions of varying intensity. Heart and lung efficiency. Synonymous with aerobic workouts.

Energy: Pick-up, get up and go, drive. Food provides calories, which provide chemical energy to produce muscle contraction and heat.

Ergogenic Aids: Anything that increases your ability to work or do exercise.

Essential Fat: Body fat crucial to body function. It is not healthy to lose so much weight and fat that you dip into this reserve.

Estrogen: Our major female sex hormone. Until menopause, estrogen acts like exercise to prevent heart attacks.

Exercise: Physical activity that burns calories. Workouts are aerobic and/or anaerobic.

Extension: Moving your arm, leg or body back to normal position after going through flexion.

EZ-Curl Barbell: A cambered (bent) weight-training bar for arm exercises.

Fartlik Training: Interval training, alternating sessions of power exercise with endurance exercise or rest. Effective for burning calories while also developing strength.

Fast-Twitch Muscle: Power muscle fiber that contracts and fatigues fast.

Fat: One of the three major food-energy nutrients. Body tissue that most of us want to get rid of!

Femininity: Being born a woman.

Flex: Showing your muscle by contracting it hard.

Flexibility: Range of motion in your joints. Flexibility is limited by tight connective tissues.

Flexion: Moving your arm, leg or body from anatomical position so that your muscle insertion moves closer to its origin.

Forced Reps: The last few repetitions in a set, assisted by a partner.

Free Weights: As opposed to weight machines, barbells, dumbbells and weights.

Frequency: How often you work out.

Fructose: A sweet fruit sugar. Also found in honey.

Gastrocnemius: A calf muscle. Your gastrocnemius is a white fiber, power muscle.

Giant Sets: A series of 4–6 exercises for the same body part, done in one of my circuit workouts.

Glucose: A simple blood sugar used for energy.

Glutes: Your rear-end muscles—your gluteus maximus, medius and minimus.

Glycemic Index: A measure of how readily and fast carbohydrates break down into their simple sugars in your bloodstream.

Glycogen: Stored muscle sugar for energy.

Golgi Tendon Organ: A complex in your muscle that monitors muscle and tendon tension, which inhibits contraction if it gets too high.

Hack Squat: Squats holding a bar behind your legs or using a special hack squat machine. Also called sissy squats.

Oops. Now that's a stretch for your inner-thigh adductors and hamstrings.

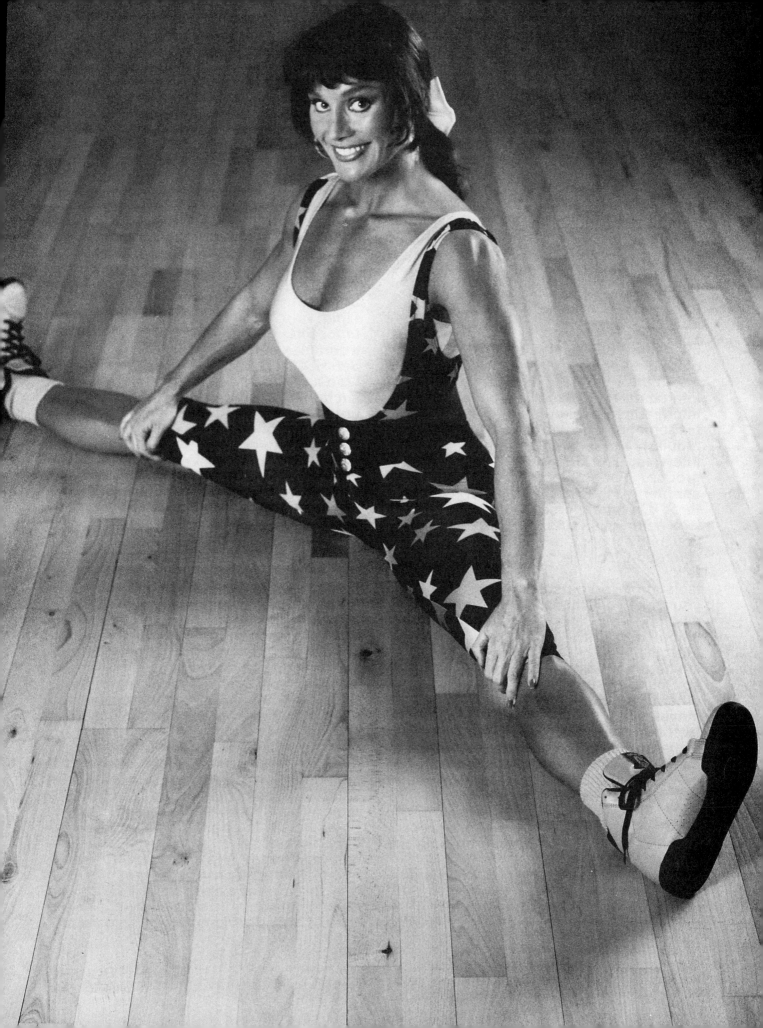

Hamstrings: Muscles in the back of your upper thighs.

HDL: High-density lipoproteins. Your good cholesterol. Exercise increases HDL levels.

Hemoglobin: A molecule that carries and releases oxygen in your blood. Women have less hemoglobin than men.

Holistic Workouts: A broad range of repetitions to work every part of your muscle cell.

Hyperplasia: Growth through splitting muscle fibers.

Hypers: Short for hyperextension. An exercise for your lower- and middle-back extensors.

Hypertrophy: Increased muscle size.

Insulin: A hormone that helps regulate sugar levels.

Intensity: Your level of effort. The amount of weight you use relative to your absolute maximum.

Intercostals: Muscles between your ribs.

Intermediate Workout: Workouts designed for someone who has trained correctly and regularly for six months to a year.

Intervals: Working out in segments or groups. For instance, a 60-yard-dash sprinter who, as part of his workout, does three 60s interspersed with three 100s.

Isokinetic Workouts: Workouts in which you train at constant velocities, without acceleration. You need special machines for this.

Isolation Workouts: Workouts in which you make your muscle work harder by positioning your limb in an anti-gravity position with little help from assistance muscles.

Isometric Workouts: Workouts in which you contract your muscles against each other or against fixed objects. There's no movement.

Isotonic Workouts: Free-weight and machine workouts in which your muscles contract, change length and tension, and move weights at varying speeds. Another name for free-weight training.

Joint: Where bones come together, joined by ligaments and connective tissues. Your elbow joint "joins" your humerus, ulna and radius.

Kinesiology: The study of human movement.

Lactate (Lactic Acid): A by-product of intense exercise which can be re-converted from being a fatigue product back to an energy source.

Lat Machine Pull-Down: The main exercise for your upper-body latissimus muscles.

LBM: Lean body mass.

LDL: Low-density lipoproteins. Your bad cholesterol. Exercise lowers LDL levels.

Leg Curl: The key exercise for your hamstring muscles.

Leg Extension: The key exercise for your quadriceps muscles.

Leg Press: A major exercise for your thighs, glutes and hips.

Lifting Belt: A 4–6″ leather belt worn around your waist for heavy lifting.

Ligament: Fibrous band that connects bones.

Lipid: Another name for fats in your blood.

Lipoproteins: In reference to cholesterol, a complex of fat and protein in your blood. See HDL and LDL.

Liposuction: Surgical removal of fat using suctioning.

Lordosis: A pronounced arch in your lower back that can lead to back pain.

LSD Workouts: Long, slow distance training to burn fat and develop cardiovascular condition.

Lunge: An exercise for your glutes, quadriceps, hip flexors and hamstrings. I also have an exercise known as the Cory Lunge.

Maximum Oxygen Uptake: Your ability to metabolize oxygen to energy. Cross-country skiers and marathon runners have the highest uptakes (also called VO2 max).

Mesomorph: A naturally muscular person with an average-to-large bone frame.

Metabolism: Using food to produce energy for all your body processes.

METS: Short for metabolic equivalents. Physiologists use this measurement to standardize energy expenditure in different forms of work.

Minerals: Substances important for normal growth and metabolism, such as calcium and iron.

Muscle: Special tissue that contracts to move your limbs. The average person's body weight is approximately 35–45 percent muscle!

Muscle-Bound: This used to erroneously mean tight muscles or lack of flexibility due to large muscles. Now it is a colloquialism meaning well built.

Muscle Pull: A strain or slight muscle tear,

most likely near the muscle attachment.

Muscle Tone: A state of heightened muscle tension or readiness. Increased ability to contract your muscles. Being in shape. Buffed. Looking good.

Muscularity: The size and definition of your muscles.

Myofibril: The individual muscle fiber. Many myofibrils make up a muscle.

Negative Workouts: Workouts in which you resist with your muscles while lowering weights. The eccentric phase of exercise.

Nitrogen Balance: The ratio of protein intake to excretion. Positive nitrogen balance is taking in more protein than your body uses and excretes. Losing more protein than you take in is negative nitrogen balance. This happens in illness and heavy training.

Obesity: Too mucy body fat. In women, having 40 percent or more body fat is obesity.

Olympic Lifting: Weight-lifting competition in the snatch and clean and jerk.

Overload: Increasing the weights you lift. Making your workouts harder.

Overtraining: Too much heavy training, too often, so you exceed your recovery ability. Also called burn-out.

Remember when Oprah Winfrey wheeled out pounds of fat on her TV show? Chicken skin may taste good, but it's all fat. Wheel it out of your life!

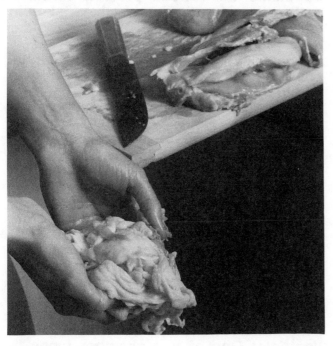

Peaking: Progressing your workouts over time to reach your physical pinnacle on the day of competition.

Pecs: Your chest pectoral muscles. Your pecs are subdivided into sternal and clavicular fibers.

Periodization Workouts: Workouts in which you divide your training into monthly and yearly cycles for endurance, strength, power and skill.

Physique: Body build.

Plyometric Workouts: Workouts with exercises where you perform a concentric (positive) contraction immediately following an eccentric (negative) contraction. Bounding and depth-jumping off boxes are examples.

Polyunsaturated Fat: A fat that is usually liquid at room temperature. Better for your health than saturated fats.

Posing: Bodybuilders artfully showing their musculature in competition to a coordinated routine set to music.

Power: Exerting force over a distance per unit time. The ability to move your limbs or objects quickly.

Power Lifting: Squat, bench press and deadlift competition.

PRE: Progressive resistance exercise.

Pre-Exhaustion Workout: Workout in which you work a muscle to failure, then work it again with assisting muscles by doing a different exercise.

Pronation: Turning your palms down. Also turning your ankles in.

Proportion: Balanced muscle development.

Protein: One of three basic food/energy groups with fats and carbohydrates. Protein and carbohydrates provide about four calories per gram when burned for energy, while fats provide over nine calories!

Pump: Muscle congestion from exercise.

Push/Pull Workouts: Workouts in which you work your muscles that "pull" (lats and biceps) with your muscles that "push" (triceps, deltoids and pectorals).

Pyramid Workout: Workouts in which you progressively increase your exercise weights and lower your repetitions. Also, progressively decreasing your weights and increasing your reps.

Quads: Four muscles in your thighs that extend your lower leg at the knee joint.

Rectus Abdominis: An abdominal muscle that flexes your torso forward.

Rectus Femoris: Your main thigh (quadricep) muscle that flexes your hip and helps extend your lower leg.

Red Muscle Fiber: Endurance muscle that contracts and fatigues slowly. Called slow-twitch fiber.

Rep: Lifting a weight one time is one repetition.

Rest Period: The time of inactivity between sets of exercise.

ROM: Range of motion. Degrees of flexibility in your joints.

Routine: Your organized exercise schedule.

SAID: Specific adaptation to imposed demands. Your muscles, heart and lungs will adapt to the type of program you do.

Sarcomere: The unit of contraction within your muscle.

Sarcoplasm: The fluid surrounding your muscle cell nucleus. Sarcoplasmic proteins increase in size and number with exercise.

Saturated Fat: Fat that is solid at room temperature. Saturated fats (such as butter) are believed to be more detrimental to your heart than polyunsaturated fats.

Scapulae: Your shoulder blades.

Serratus: Muscles that cover your upper ribs.

Set: A group of repetitions.

Shape: Your unique combination of bone structure, body-fat distribution and muscle.

Smith Machine: A machine with a weight bar attached to glide rods. Athletes use the Smith Machine for safety and muscle isolation.

Soleus: A calf muscle. Your soleus is a red fiber, endurance muscle.

Somatotyping: Classifying your physique by a combination of ectomorphy, mesomorphy and endomorphy.

Split Workouts: Workouts in which you work upper body one day and your lower body on your next training day. Or, working different body parts on different days.

Spot Reduction: The myth that you can reduce body fat in only one specific area without taking off some fat everywhere.

Spotters: People who assist you in finishing an exercise if you can't do it on your own.

Spot Toning: Concentrating on one area of your body to increase muscle tone. Like doing sit-ups for your abdominals.

Squat: Also called knee bend, this is the most effective and popular lower-body exercise to strengthen your thighs and lower back.

Storage Fat: Fat that protects and cushions your internal organs, providing energy.

Strength: Developing or exerting maximum force such as in a one-rep maximum in the bench press.

Stretching: Moving your limbs to a point where there's slight discomfort in muscle and supporting connective tissues. Holding this point is static stretching.

Stretch Marks: Slight tears in your skin caused by gaining weight (fat or muscle) too fast. The excess weight stretches your skin and exceeds the momentary pliability of your skin, leaving a scar.

Stretch Reflex: A neurological reaction whereby a muscle contraction will be more powerful if it is immediately preceded by a slight, quick stretch of the same muscles that will be used in the contraction.

Striations: Definition of muscle so extreme (with low fat) that large muscle-fiber bundles can be observed under your skin.

Supersets: Doing a set of one exercise immediately followed by a set of a different exercise. These are usually done with antagonistic muscle groups.

Superwraps: Special knee bands to aid squatting power and protect your knees.

Supination: Turning your palms up or your ankles out.

Supplements: Various protein, carbohydrate, vitamin and mineral mixes taken in addition to, or instead of, your regular food.

Symmetry: The structure of your frame. The proportion of your torso and limbs in bodybuilding competition.

Tendon: Fibrous tissue connecting muscle to bone.

Tension: The amount of force developed by a muscle when it contracts.

Testosterone: The major male sexual hormone.

Triceps: The large three-headed muscle on the back of your upper arms that performs elbow and shoulder joint extension.

Triglycerides: Fat particles in your blood.

Valsalva: Holding your breath as you exert maximum force. Avoid this at all times. Do not hold your breath when you lift weights.

Vascularity: Prominent veins because of dehydration and low body fat.

Ventricle: One of two chamber types in

your heart. Your left ventricle pumps blood through your aorta for general circulation.

Vertebrae: Your spinal bones.

Vitamins: Necessary cofactors in metabolism which are either water or fat soluble. For example, vitamin A is fat soluble, vitamin C is water soluble.

Volume: The total amount of work in your workouts. For example, the number of exercises, sets, reps and weight in your workout.

Warm-Up: Calisthenics, stretching or a sustained activity to elevate tissue and blood temperature before your workout.

Weight Lifting: Technically, weight lifting is synonymous with Olympic-style lifting (snatch and clean and jerk). However, like weight training, it has become a generic term for sports training, bodybuilding, power lifting, or any form of pumping iron.

White Muscle Fiber: Power muscle that contracts and fatigues quickly. Also called fast-twitch fiber.

Working to Failure: Performing your reps on a set until total fatigue.

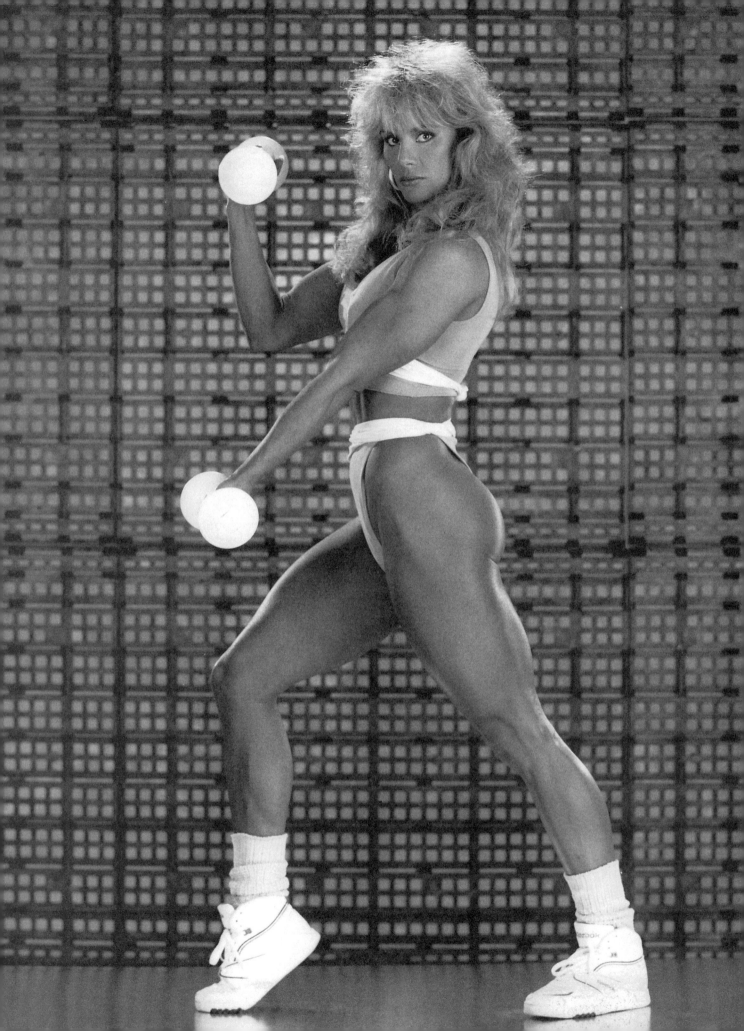

3
STARTING WEIGHT-TRAINING WORKOUTS

A new workout is exciting but confusing. What do you want to accomplish? Your first priority is setting realistic goals for your lifestyle. If you are a busy executive, a parent of five children, a construction worker, of if you travel a lot, your workouts should be different from someone with a lot of spare time and energy.

Most women want to drop fat and improve their shape and sex appeal. Men usually want to drop fat too, plus build muscle. The rules for shaping and toning are basic. If you are overweight with too much fat, cut calories by eliminating fatty foods and begin an exercise program that you can stay with. Your workout program must include a mix of endurance and body-toning weight exercises.

On the other hand, if you are skinny and underweight, you have to eat more good food, particularly good carbohydrates, and follow a good weight-training workout. Endurance exercises can wait. Don't do too

Weight training, sports and aerobics are part of Cory's workout. Get the body you want!

many aerobic workouts when you are trying to gain muscle weight. You will be burning too many calories.

No matter which goal you have, start slowly. Rome wasn't built in a day and you can't build your body into a muscular, fit empire in a day either.

WHERE TO WORK OUT

You have a couple of choices: your home, a commercial gym, a school or a YMCA. Don't be afraid of free weights, bars and dumbbells. Use free weights. They're versatile and more effective than many machines. Machines should supplement free weights and in some cases, machines will be all you can use.

At home, you're limited. You can do a lot of exercises with dumbbells, a multi-purpose weight bench and a barbell set, or with handy home machines. At a club you can do more exercises with more variety, socialize and take aerobics classes. Do you like the social atmosphere of a gym? With people, more equipment and a change in venue, workouts are less boring. Clubs can be expensive and some people are too self-conscious to go into a gym; they would rather shape up at home first.

If you join a gym, take advantage of everything it offers for workout variety. Pick a gym that fits your budget and is close to home or work. The gym should have instructors to answer questions or lend training spots and advice. Your best source for learning at a gym? Your eyes! Watch some of the accomplished people training to learn correct exercise techniques.

You can get a good workout at home. It's not important *where* you train, it's important *that* you train. It's time to get off the dime and turn your body into a hundred-dollar gold piece.

WHAT TO DO

Don't follow Bo Jackson's workout! If you were a student pilot, would you feel comfortable starting out at the controls of a 747-400? If you did, the passengers could be in trouble. Start with a workout you can handle. Your first workouts should be fairly easy, leaving you energetic and refreshed when you finish. Your workout should be basic, nothing fancy, no plyometric workouts or cross training.

Work your entire body in one session, each day, three alternating days a week. Do that for the first three months before trying anything more demanding with weights. With beginning endurance or cardiovascular workouts, you can work out every day, but do moderate work, a 30-minute walk, for instance. I'll have plenty of workouts later!

Technique is critical to success. With most weight-training exercises, start your first few workouts with just an empty bar and dumbbells to learn good form.

Warm up! Stretch, jog in place, do calisthenics or warm up with a short stay in a hot tub or whirlpool. A lot of experienced athletes take a warm shower immediately before training and do pre-exercises and stretching, as well as starting with light weights and high repetitions.

Don't overdo it! If you do too much too soon, you delay progress by overtraining.

Good food, rest, sleep and day-to-day recovery are important. You grow and get better through adaptation to harder workouts. Both workout and recovery are important to success. If you slight either, you slight yourself.

HOW OFTEN SHOULD YOU TRAIN? HOW MANY SETS AND REPS?

Coax, don't blast, your body. After three months of technique work with light weights and basic exercises, you can try more complicated exercises. Even if you are super-enthusiastic, train only three days per week if you are just starting. Three months go by quickly.

For each body part, 1–3 exercises are fine. Do 2–4 sets per exercise. For your upper-body exercises, 8–12 repetitions are a good base. For your lower-body work, 10–20 repetitions are best. There are a couple of exceptions, like calves and abdominals, where you should do more reps.

Always refer to my "Mouse in a Maze" chapter if you have questions about terminology. A set is a series of repetitions. Doing the exercise once is one repetition. If you do 10 curls, rest, then do 10 more curls, you have done two sets of 10 reps, written 2 × 10.

SOME TRAINING SPECIFICS

As I mentioned earlier, beginners must get used to new exercises before piling on tons of weight. Style is more important at first. It's not *how much* you lift, it's *how* you lift! Plus, by using light weights when you could use heavier weights, you'll avoid muscle soreness which is part of every new exercise program. Soreness is your body telling you it's being worked!

Muscle soreness from a new program usually lasts 24–72 hours. If it lasts longer than this, you might have strained something and you should lay off training; if the soreness gets substantially worse or doesn't go away, see your doctor. If you use light weights at first and break in slowly, soreness won't be a problem.

In general, beginners can follow this simple program:

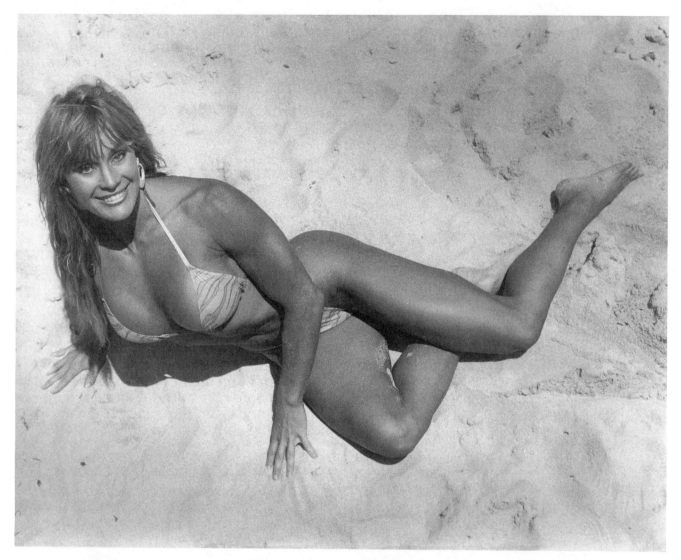

Don't worry about your bikini bod next summer. Train with weights and you'll look fine.

Week One

Do one or two sets of each exercise. Do two exercises per body part. Do 8–12 reps for all upper-body exercises. Do 10–20 reps for all lower-body exercises. Train three alternate days in the first week.

Weeks Two and Three:

Progress to at least two sets of each exercise using the same repetitions. Continue to do two exercises per body part. Counting your chest, shoulders, arms, abdominals, back, thighs and calves, that's 14 exercises per day, which is enough.

After three weeks, gradually increase your workout weights, exercises and sets. There is no formula or accurate percentage of maximum to determine how much weight you should use in your exercises. Everyone has different strength and endurance levels. Weight is relative.

In fact, as simple as it may seem, the best way to determine your weights is by trial and error. If you're doing 8–12 reps, you should fail somewhere around 11 or 12. You shouldn't fail at seven or 14! The trial-and-error method is specific. When you exceed the upper repetition number, add weight.

I include beginning, intermediate and advanced levels in my specific workouts. Developing strength, power, sports ability and endurance is hard enough without being confused about them. Don't be confused. Here are some guidelines:

1. To develop power (the ability to generate muscle force rapidly), 1–5 repetitions are best. Olympic weight lifters are powerful athletes, and they usually perform less than five reps on all exercises. See my sports workouts.

2. For strength (maximum force), 1–8 repetitions are best.

3. For optimum muscle size, professional bodybuilders do a variety of repetitions. However, the majority of them do 8–15 repetitions on every set.

4. For muscle endurance, do 20–50 reps with little rest between sets. High reps are hard, but these workouts are great for endurance events, such as running.

5. Professional bodybuilders do 4–10 sets of *each* exercise. That's a lot, but they

have been at it for years and they have adapted to these workouts.

6. Regardless if you are a beginner, intermediate or advanced trainee, warm up and cool down. Before your workout, do about 10 minutes of stretching, jogging in place or calisthenics. Stretch, walk or bike after your workout to cool down.

WORKOUT EXERCISE SPEED

Don't explode and sling your weights around. You will not develop faster by training this way, but you might injure yourself. Use a steady, slow exercise cadence and good technique.

REST TIME

There isn't any exact time to rest between sets. However, to burn fat and develop endurance and definition, don't rest very long between sets, maybe 30–60 seconds. Or if

Cory has to "lounge" in the sun for professional photo shoots, but too much of ol' sol is not good for your skin.

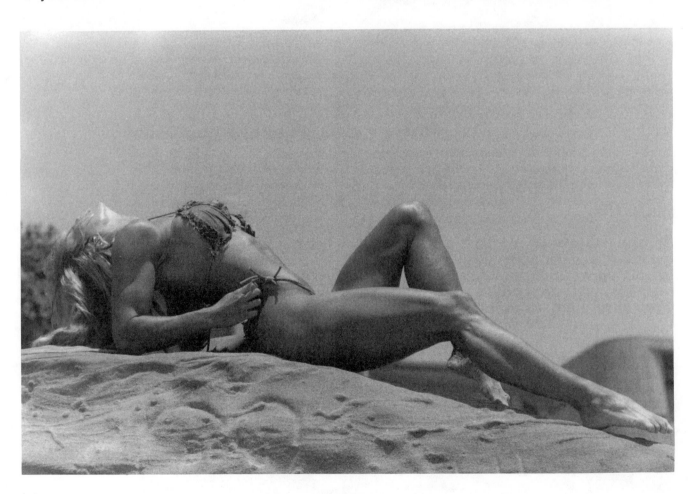

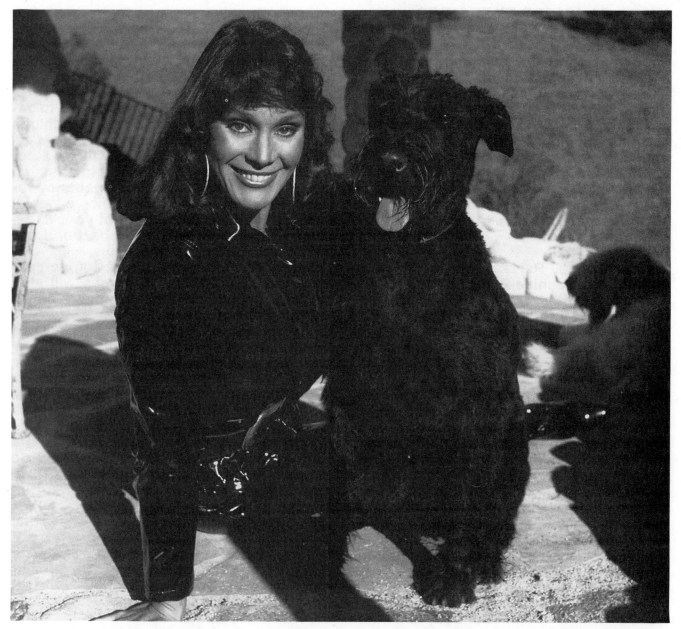

Overlooking the hills from her backyard gazebo, Cory pauses with pal Bolaro, her Giant Schnauzer.

you do a circuit workout, try not to rest at all between sets or exercises. On the other hand, if you are interested in strength and muscle size, rest longer to lift heavier weights, maybe 90 seconds to three minutes.

Work big muscles before smaller muscles. If you just did three months of squats, bench presses and lat machine pulldowns, you'd improve in shape and strength because these exercises work big muscle groups. An hour of squatting is better than an hour of wrist curls!

A BREATH OF FRESH AIR

If you're confused about how to breathe during lifting, just don't hold your breath; breathe naturally. For safety, with heavy lifting exhale on the exertion part. In the bench press, for example, breathe in while lowering the weight and breathe out when you push it up.

It's a good idea to wear a weight-lifting belt for support when working out, especially when you do squats and presses.

MY 10 FAVORITE EXERCISES

There are a lot of weight-training exercises and you can't possibly do all of them. You shouldn't try! Some are more effective than others. Some are easy, some aren't. In my workouts, I repeat many exercises for different sports or different shaping/toning workouts. My 10 favorite and most effective exercises are:

1. Squat
2. Leg Extension
3. Leg Curl
4. Crunch
5. Donkey Raise
6. Lat Machine Pull-Down
7. Dumbbell Curl
8. Tricep Push-Down
9. Incline Dumbbell Press
10. Hyperextension

CORY'S RULES

If you are a beginner, don't copy a champion's workout. You need time to adapt to tougher workouts and this takes gradual conditioning.

To learn brain surgery, you wouldn't operate for two minutes a month or for 16 hours a day. You'd be too inexperienced if you operated only two minutes a month. Operating 16 hours a day would cause fatigue and mistakes.

Your brain has a limited ability to store and learn information. Your body has a limited, built-in ability to develop and change too.

If you lifted a one-pound dumbbell continuously, you would probably get weaker instead of stronger. Without time to recuperate, even light-weight exercise would cause overtraining, whether you're an accomplished athlete or a weekend warrior.

Here are a few simple rules to follow:

Frequency/Intensity/Volume/Duration

You have to work out often enough to progress. This is called workout frequency. If you work out super hard and heavy, but only train twice a year, you won't make many gains because your workout frequency is too low. With my earlier example with the one-pound dumbbell, if you lift this weight all the time, you also won't progress because your frequency is too high for your recovery ability. Your workout frequency depends on your capacity to recover, diet, sleep, job, health, athletic ability, attitude and lifestyle.

Work out hard enough to force a response. This is called workout intensity. If you work out with the right frequency for your body (let's say, three times a week), but you lift only 20 percent of your capability, your progress won't be good because your intensity is too low.

If you lift (or attempt to lift) 100 percent of your capacity, your progress will also be poor. In fact, you will probably be injured most of the time!

You must do enough work. This is called volume. Let's say your frequency is okay and your intensity is right. For example, when you work your chest, you use 60–75 percent of your maximum capabilities. However, if in your whole workout you do only one set for your chest, your progress will be slow since you need to do more sets (higher volume). Likewise, if you do 100 sets per workout, you'll make little progress. You'll overtrain, get bored and injure yourself.

Work out long enough. If you have the right intensity and volume and work out the correct number of days, it's better to train for 45–75 minutes than 15 minutes or three hours. After about an hour, you get bored and your energy drops. The same is true with any sport.

What about doing one set to failure with maximum weight? I don't buy that. You need more sets, even though one set is 100 percent better than no sets!

The rules are really easy in practice even if I lost you in the translation. PRE (progressive resistance exercise) might explain things better.

PRE

Progressive resistance exercise underlies all workouts. To progress, overload your muscles in a disciplined, progressive way. Say you could bench-press 30 pounds 20 times when you start. If you bench press

20 pounds for two sets of 20 reps every other day for a year, you develop some muscle tone and endurance in your chest, shoulder and arm muscles. However, you won't get much stronger or larger, and you might get bored.

However, if you gradually, progressively increase your bench weight, chances are you will do three or more sets of 20 reps with well over 60 pounds after one year. Not only will you have more tone and endurance, but you will be stronger with larger muscles. Because muscles get denser and stronger and you lose fat as you gain muscle, you might be only 1–2 pounds heavier after the year of workouts.

If over that same year you do three sets of bench presses every other day, but work out with heavier weights for 8–10 reps instead of 20, you would gain endurance, size and *more* strength.

The best way to keep building muscle size and strength is to change your workouts frequently. There's no rule, of course; you can stay on any workout program as long as you progress. After the technique break-in period, beginner and intermediate periods, or after your first year of training, you'll have the knowledge to change your routine for the better. By changing your workouts, your body does not become accustomed to routines. Stay progressive.

CONCENTRATION

You can't achieve anything unless you figure out what you want. Dreams are important, but sweat and inspiration make your

Look what washed ashore!

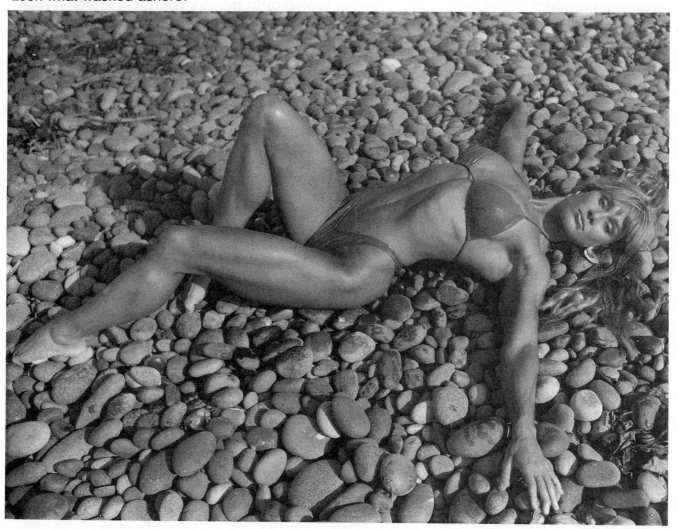

body fit. Here are some keys to concentration and focus:

1. Be realistic. Everyone can make gains; not everyone can be an Olympic champion. Do your best but set realistic goals and don't set new ones until you have reached your old goals.

2. Be realistic but don't limit yourself. Always believe you have unlimited potential and then strive to reach it!

3. Be positive. Don't get down on your present condition. Look around and you'll see suffering and ill health. You're wealthier than the richest man alive if you have good health and he doesn't. Accentuate positive things in your life. Eliminate negative emotions.

4. Be disciplined. Stick to your workout time and schedule like beef to a rib. Your workout is a business plan. Stay true to your workout days, sets and reps.

5. If you lack motivation, recruit a workout partner. Choose someone who is serious about working out and develop a good relationship.

6. Focus on your workouts. Don't gab and weaken your focus through conversation. Don't be a jerk in the gym, but stick to business.

7. Think about your sets, reps and weights. Focus on your muscle action.

8. Picture yourself in top shape, slim and strong. Eventually, with the right workouts, you will be!

REST AND SLEEP

Sleep and rest are as important as diet in your quest for super shape. If you're thin and trying to gain weight or muscle, cut back outside activities. Put your energy into your weight-training workouts. If you have a fast metabolism and cannot gain weight (overweight people should have this problem!), never walk when you can ride, never stand when you can sit!

To get more sleep, learn to relax. Stop smoking and drinking and cut back on caffeine. The easiest way to get rest and sleep is to get on a fixed schedule. If you have the opportunity, a 30–60-minute nap in midday is worth about three hours of sleep at night. Sleep requirements vary; most people need 7–9 hours of sleep. Go to sleep and get up at the same time each day.

Don't exercise within 2–3 hours of bedtime. Exercise keeps you up. Don't have a big meal within three hours of bedtime and don't argue or debate before bedtime. Your mind will be working overtime. Your body can't relax when your mind isn't off duty.

You can't get your workouts under control until you get your sleep and rest under control.

HOW LONG WILL IT TAKE?

You will make gains fast if you work out right. You might not notice it because workouts are cumulative and they add slowly. After a week of workouts, you will have an awareness of your muscles. You will have better muscle control. This is good muscle tone.

Before long, maybe at the three- or four-month period, friends will begin making statements, "Lost weight, Sue?" or "Lookin' good, Bill. Did you go on vacation or something?" At 6–10 months, the comments get more specific. "Wendy, how's those muscles coming?" Or, "Been pumping a little iron, or what?" You'd be surprised, you might not notice your changes, but others will!

Just as all of this is certain, you won't look like a professional bodybuilder in six months. Most of the competitors in the magazines have been training for over 10 years! Be patient, you'll get there!

WHAT IF YOU'RE OVER 35?

There's nothing mystical about the age 35. Many people over 35 act 20 and are in very good shape. However, there are changes in your body after age 20 or 25 or so, and by 35 to 40, most people are stiffer and not in as good shape as they were 10 or 15 years earlier. Still, it's encouraging that people in middle age (middle age to me is

Children can exercise, too, but nothing strenuous, and games and play are better than organized sports when they are young.

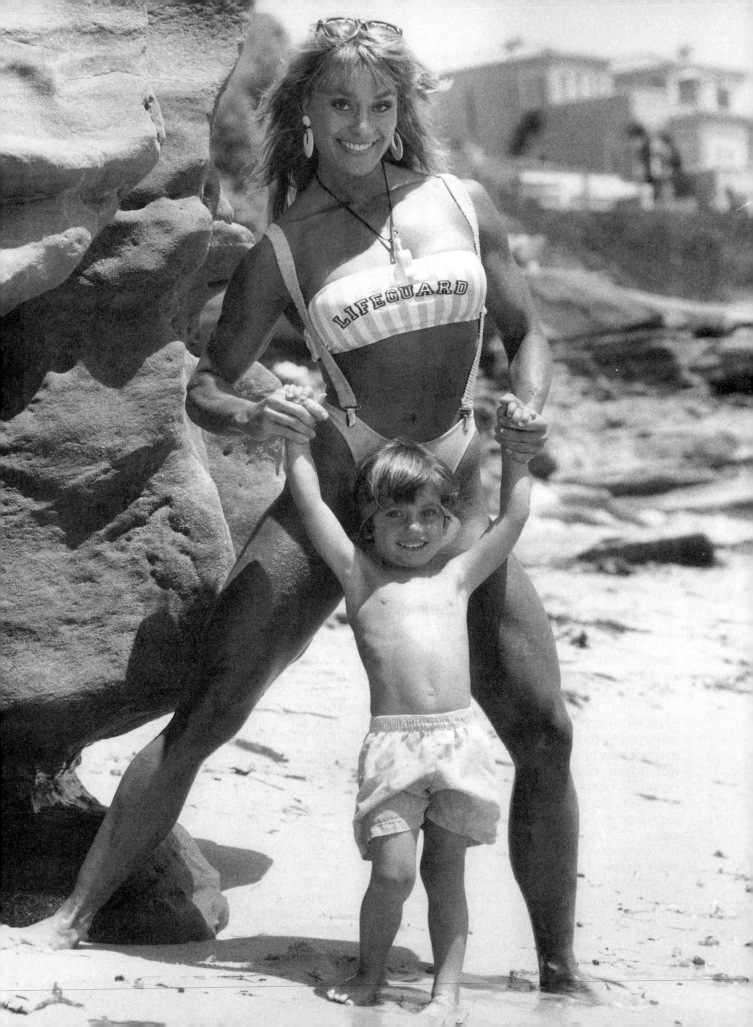

45 to 65) can "get back" their shape of their late teens and early twenties with weight-training workouts. In fact, at that age, if you have never done weights, you can make yourself fitter than you were at 20.

However, there are some things you should do differently if you are over 35 and inactive:

1. It is imperative that you be examined by your doctor before starting an exercise program.

2. Spend more time warming up and cooling down.

3. Other than during your beginning stage, you *cannot* do as many exercises or sets of exercise as when you were younger because recovery is slower.

4. Because joint fluid diminishes with age, skip the squat, deadlift, power clean, T-bar row, bent-over row and behind-the-neck press exercises. Other exercises are okay.

5. Pay more attention to your diet. Eat more fruits and vegetables and much less fat.

6. Do aerobic endurance exercise, which is very important for your heart.

Most of my workout principles apply, but I do have a special workout for those of you over 35 and just starting.

WHAT ABOUT KIDS?

Doctors pooh-pooh weight training for kids until age 16 or so. You have sensitive growth centers in your long bones and vertebrae until you are mature, which, as far as bones are concerned, usually takes place by age 18.

Weight training does *not* stunt your growth and if done correctly, is in no way damaging to kids. In fact, your teen years are an excellent time to start because of hormonal changes favoring growth and development. If you do certain exercises and you do them heavy, before you have matured, you may damage some soft tissues.

However, you can still work out, first with nonweight exercises (like push-ups, sprints and pull-ups) and then with non-weight-bearing resistance exercises. Because of soft tissue growth activity, kids under 16 should *not* do heavy squats, deadlifts, overhead presses or heavy max-

imum lifts for less than six repetitions (that's weight lifting and should be avoided).

Do a supervised, varied weight program of groups of all the other good exercises. Kids should be able to do 10–15 reps of almost all exercises. However, avoid maximum lifts. Kids need an endurance/strength base to build on. You don't need to be a teenage Hercules and then develop a bad back when you are 35.

I have included a workout for kids!

NO ROOM AT THE INN FOR THE PHYSICALLY CHALLENGED?

It bothers me that exercise programs are made for everybody but the physically challenged. I guess that's like the world in general, isn't it? If you don't fit into the norm, you're out of luck. That attitude stinks and I have included a special program designed by my physical-therapist husband, Jeff.

PREGNANCY

You can work out through your seventh or eighth month, gradually tapering off as you get closer to the big date. Use your head. Needless to say, nutrition is important. You are now eating for two so you must consume enough calories and a very well-balanced diet. Don't be afraid to gain 25–35 pounds!

Both weight training and low-impact aerobics are okay. However, you should follow your obstetrician's advice on exercise and heart rates. Many doctors now feel that if you do aerobics, don't go for your maximum. Instead of going up to 70–85 percent of your maximum heart rate, 50–60 percent is better. Eliminate bounding, running and any jarring aerobics. Try stationary biking, walking and swimming instead.

Eliminate "high abdominal pressure" weight training exercises like deadlifts and squats. Correct breathing is even more important. Don't hold your breath during any exercises. Don't do any inverted leg presses or abdominal exercises where your head and heart are lower than your baby's, or where you lie flat on your back. Theoretically, this position might interfere with blood flow to your baby.

Be cautious and wise with your workouts. Baby will thank you for it!

HOW IMPORTANT IS STRETCHING?

Stretching should be fun, but done with purpose. Good flexibility not only makes you look, move and feel better, it prevents injuries.

Stretching stimulates your muscles and connective tissues. Stretching, as part of a general warm-up, helps raise your blood temperature and thins your blood. When this happens, your body becomes more elastic and this prevents injuries.

Tension and stress can be an enemy. Stretching relaxes muscles by inhibiting sensitive receptors within your muscles. Stretching tells your muscles to reduce internal tension and relax. If everyone could reduce their level of stress, they could add five years (or more) to their life.

Flexibility is individual. Some people are naturally flexible. Women are generally more flexible than men. Some people have flexible hips but tight hamstring muscles. Not everyone can get by with five minutes of stretching a day. Some people need 30 minutes a day. Begin *every* workout with a warm-up, including stretching. Include stretching in your cool-down period, too.

Use a belt or a stick to begin stretching your upper-body muscles.

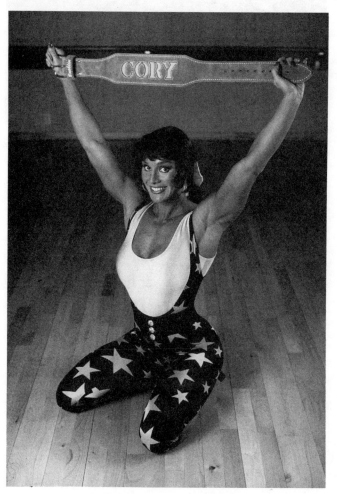

This is a full stretch of your pectoral and anterior deltoid muscles.

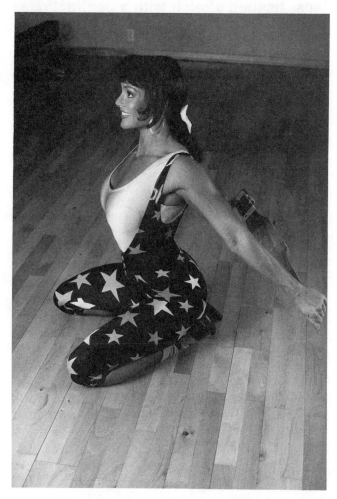

Here are my guidelines for stretching:

1. Don't force stretching. Good flexibility takes time.

2. Stretch every major muscle area including your calves, hamstrings, quadriceps, hip flexors and rotators, lower-back extensors, chest and shoulder muscles, neck, wrist and upper-back muscles. Usually, your abdominal muscles aren't tight. Instead, they're weak!

3. Don't hold your breath when you stretch.

4. Stretch statically. Don't bounce! Stretch until you feel slight discomfort in your muscles (not pain). Hold that position for five seconds, relax and repeat at least five times.

5. As you get more flexible, move farther into your range of motion. Continue to stretch statically and be patient. If you have a tight area that might be an old injury (scar tissue), stretch with a contract/relax procedure.

6. To stretch with contract/relax, you need a partner. Stretch with slight discomfort. Then contract your muscle isometrically in the opposite direction of your stretch. Your partner prevents motion, using his hands and body. Do the contract phase for five to seven seconds. Then relax. When you relax, your partner should move your limb slightly farther into the range of motion to a new point of discomfort. Repeat the procedure two or three times.

7. Stretch your hamstrings, hip flexors, pectorals, calves, lower-back extensors and shoulder area more often.

8. Skip dangerous stretches. Don't do any full-squat bouncing stretches, no hurdlers stretches, no lower-back stretches with your knees locked and legs completely straight and don't roll up and back on your neck and shoulders to stretch your lower back.

Whatever you do, don't neglect stretching.

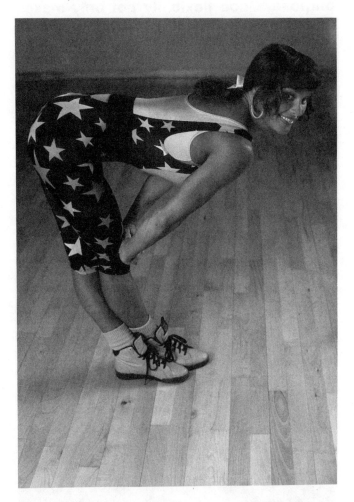

This is a pretty good way to stretch your heel cords, hamstrings and lower back extensors.

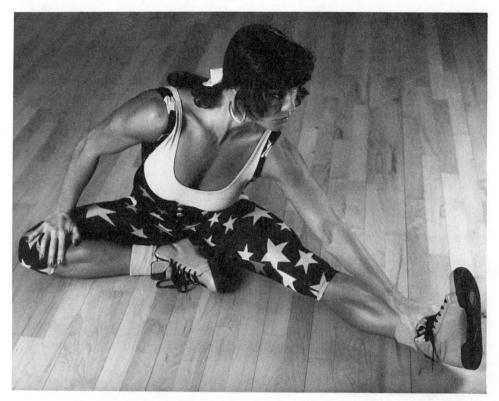

A stretch for hamstrings, heel cord and buttock muscles.

I'm not auditioning for pro wrestling, just stretching my quadriceps.

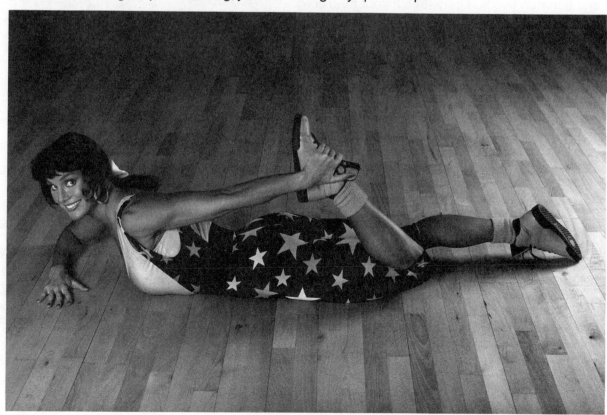

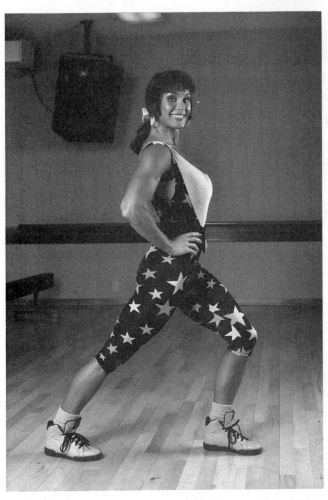

Take a march position and stretch your heel cord.

Mobilize and stretch your ankles, too.

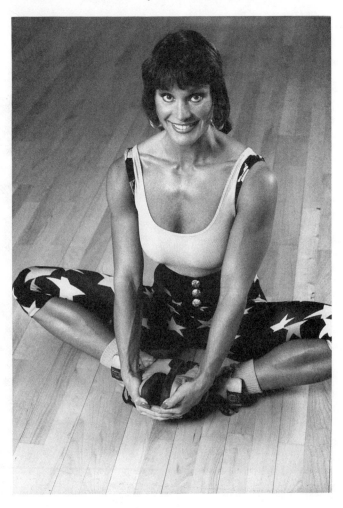

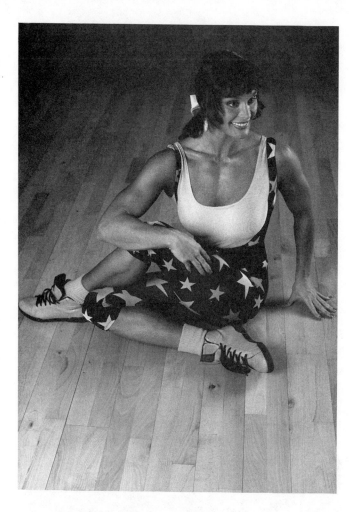

This position stretches your hip rotators.

Am I playing Hindu yoga master? No, but I am stretching my adductors and warming up my stiff neck!

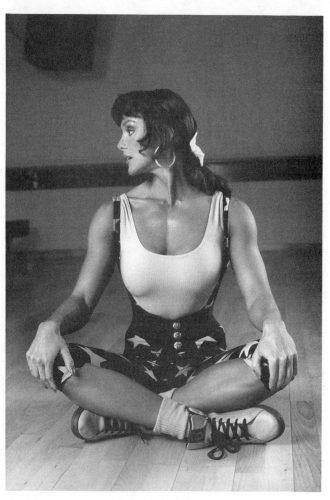

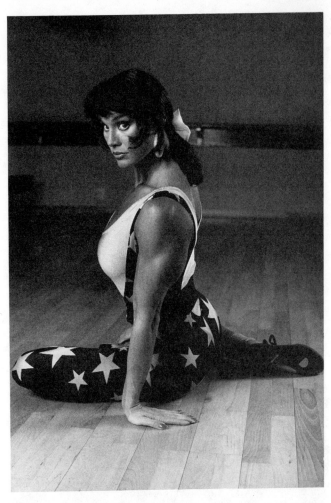

Here's a convenient way to stretch your wrist flexors.

Stretch out your wrist flexors this way, too!

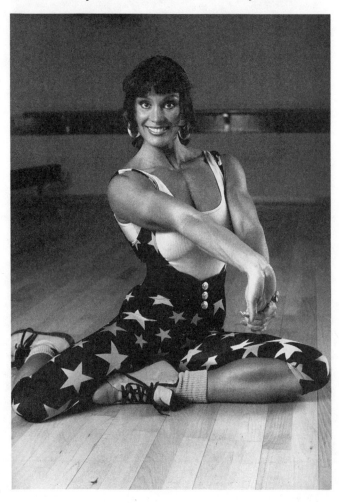

CAN YOU SPOT REDUCE?

You can spot reduce, but not exclusively. You can lose more fat from one area than another because you have more fat there to start with! You *cannot* lose fat solely from one area of your body without also losing some fat from other areas of your body, even if the amount and rate are less. In that sense, technically you can't spot reduce.

If you have normal body-fat distribution everywhere in your body except your hips and rear end, and you go on a vigorous workout program of aerobics and anaerobics plus a strict diet, you will lose fat from all over your body and you most definitely will lose *more* from your fatty areas, your hips and rear end. If you are successful in losing a lot of weight, then, in effect, you have spot reduced!

Adding to the effect of losing more fat from one area of your body than from another is spot toning. (Lord knows when you gain fat, you can gain it much more in some areas than others, so it makes sense you can also lose it at greater rates from certain areas.) A lack of muscle tone makes having too much fat even worse and, when you build up your underlying muscles, you add support and your problem area looks much better, even if you don't lose any fat there!

The semantics don't matter. Work out and eat right and even the toughest fatty problem areas can be beat and I'll show you how to do it!

MY WORKOUT TRIANGLE: WHERE DO AEROBICS FIT IN AND WHICH ONES?

Does that heading sound odd? Who would ask where do aerobics fit in when aerobics have been promulgated as the be-all and end-all for fitness and weight control? While aerobics are great for cardiovascular shape, they're not enough in the formula for total fitness, health and weight control. Weight training and nutrition make up the other sides of my workout triangle.

Aerobics, like running and cross-country skiing, are great for your heart and lungs. To a certain extent, they also tone some of your muscles and make you more flexible, enduring and strong in some areas of your body. These activities burn a lot of fat while you do them. Therefore, they help weight control. Aerobics stimulate your metabolism, but they're not enough if you have a stubborn weight problem or if you want to increase your flexibility and muscle mass.

Complete conditioning should include weight training because of all the wonderful benefits weights provide. Nutrition is a factor. If you jog and lift weights, but you eat 50 doughnuts and 30 egg yolks a week, good luck. You need to lower the fat in your diet.

All that being self-evident, which aerobics are best? The exercise format that you enjoy the most is always the best! But I think some aerobic exercises are much

You should do aerobics, and the treadmill is handy for this.

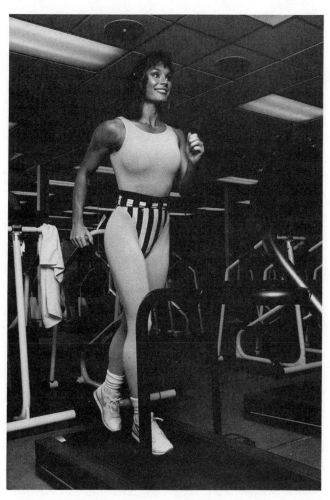

43

better than others, especially for women who have problem fat areas.

For example, many people insist swimming is the best aerobic exercise. I swam competitively for nearly 10 years. I can still swim at least 200 laps in an Olympic-size pool without stopping. So I know about swimming.

Too many people are not efficient in the water and they fight themselves when they swim. Their muscles tire out before they get a heart and lung workout. Outside, weather is sometimes a factor and in or out, you need an open lane. Some studies suggest that swimming is not as efficient as other aerobics in burning fat and losing weight. This might have something to do with cool water slowing metabolism.

A lot of women fight fatty hips, thighs and rear ends. Swimming is not the best conditioner for these areas. Compare swimming with the local toning effect from

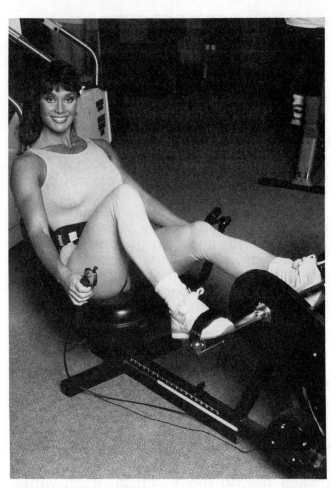

The recumbent cycle is an interesting alternative to the stationary bike.

Stair stepping works your heart aerobically and also your hip, thigh and butt muscles.

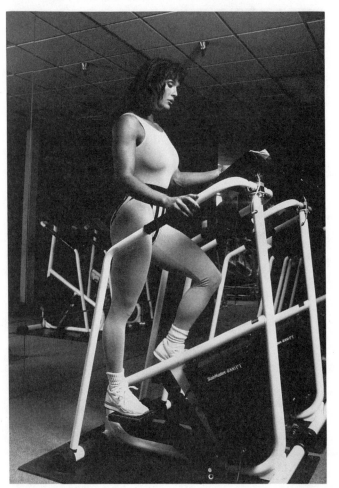

stair climbing or The Step, for instance. However, if you are a good swimmer and enjoy it, then by all means continue. If you can swim, it's good exercise and easy on your joints.

Jumping rope requires some skill too and is hard on your feet and shins. Sometimes you can't do it indoors because of lack of space or neighbors in the apartment below, or outdoors because of weather. Plus, it's boring and hard on your shoulders!

Cross-country skiing is the toughest and most invigorating aerobic exercise, but pretty tough to do in Honolulu. You could try the indoor skiing simulators. These are good because you use all-around body movement.

Jogging is famous for shin, ankle, knee and lower-back injuries and is also subject to weather, lousy drivers and irritable, property-protective dogs. However, it does produce wonderful cardiac benefits.

Indoor stationary biking and stair climbing are good exercises. Neither are subject to ornery dogs, birdbrains driving cars dangerously, potholes or sudden rainstorms. Your tires won't go flat nor will your chain derail (outdoor biking). Your shins won't ache and you won't get chlorine-infected ears (swimming).

STATIONARY BIKES

You can read the morning newspaper and watch TV while you ride. With many bikes and climbers you can program your workouts to make them more interesting. Stationary biking, though, can also be boring and in some cases with men, causes temporary groin irritation and tingling after

The stationary bike is the old standby for aerobics. Keep your heart rate in your target zone for at least 20 minutes.

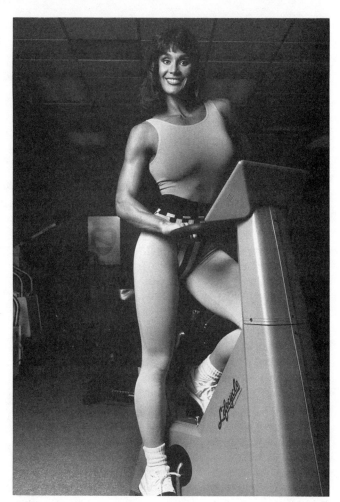

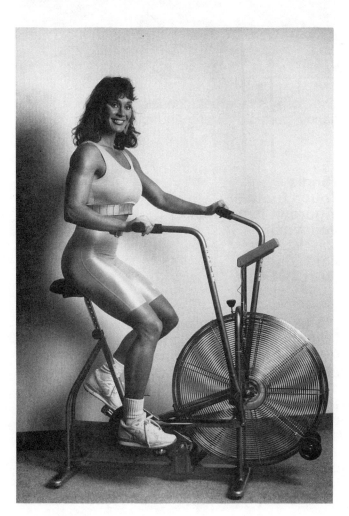

about 20 minutes. You might try the new recumbent cycles.

The bikes with special arm handles are great because you can use your arms and legs for a more efficient workout. Some bikes produce a comfortable breeze that blows backward from the front wheel. This helps cool you down during advanced aerobic workouts (there are air guards if you don't want the cooling breeze). With some bikes you can vary your protocols to match your workout ability.

THE STEP

One of the greatest new aerobic innovations is The Step. The Step is an adjustable, colorful, interlocking unit secure enough for you to do a step-up protocol. The big advantages with The Step are that you can quickly change the height of the unit and the unit is very lightweight, but strong and convenient. The Step program is a great aerobic workout and if you use hand weights or light dumbbells, you get some strength conditioning effects for your whole body with a more intense aerobic conditioning effect too. I am impressed with The Step and have developed a special aerobic/anaerobic workout video with it.

In my opinion, if you have saddlebag thighs with fat storage problems in your rear, the best indoor aerobic workout is with The Step, the stationary bike and stair climbing. For real outdoor activity, hill walking can't be beat. Hill walking elevates your heart rate and provides local muscle toning. Combined with weight-training circuits and low-fat nutrition, hill walking is tops!

My point is this: For complete workouts, do aerobics along with weights, but vary your aerobics. You'll have more fun while getting in shape.

Popular Recreational Exercise Activities and Calories Used per Hour for a 175-Pound Man (Average)

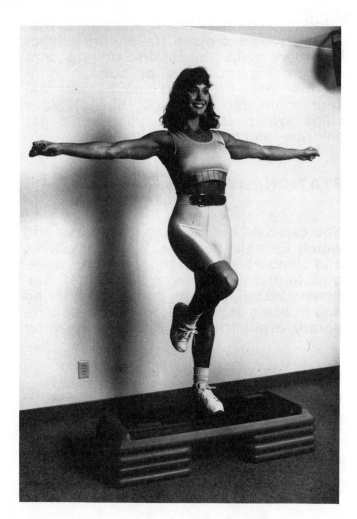

The step is a great conditioning device. Very handy, portable, strong and functional.

Archery	200
Baseball/Softball	275
Basketball (pickup)	300
Bowling	200
Circuit weight training	350
Cross-country skiing	650
Fast walking	280
Formal aerobics class	375–500
Free calisthenics	275
Golf (walking, carrying clubs)	300
Hiking on uneven terrain	275
Hill walking	325
Jet skiing	275
Light stretching	100
Martial arts workout	325
Mountain biking	375
Mountain rock climbing	500
Racquetball	400
Road biking	295
Rope jumping	400
Rough-water rafting	300
Rowing	300
Sailing	250
Skating	325
Stair climbing	340
Stationary biking	350
Step classes	300–500
Swimming (endurance)	325
Swimming (sprints)	375
Tennis	300
Touch football	325
Vigorous fast dancing	400
Volleyball	300

INJURIES

It's likely that you will get an injury here and there, no matter how safe your fitness workout is. Recreational tennis enthusiasts get tennis elbow, swimmers get sore shoulders and runners have problems with their knees and lower back. I imagine that everyone, at some time in their life, has sprained or turned an ankle.

The key is to never let an acute injury become chronic! If an injury is bad and lingers, you have already waited too long. Of course, you can't run to your doctor with every little nagging pain, but if you hear a "snap" or tearing, if you have an unexplained loss of strength (even if you don't feel pain), or if you get swelling or turn black and blue, it's important to see your doctor.

Most injuries are minor, a slight muscle pull, for example. But, even minor injuries need treatment, especially rest! Here is a short primer for injuries:

1. When you suffer an injury, stop working out and don't try to work through it. This is always a mistake.

2. If possible, elevate the injured area to minimize swelling and internal bleeding.

3. Apply ice to the area right away. Ice will help minimize swelling and bleeding. However, don't apply ice directly to your skin or you could suffer an ice burn. Instead, wrap ice in a bag or a thin towel, then apply it.

4. With any audible popping, tearing or snapping, see a doctor as soon as possible. Don't move the area around until you can see a doctor. If the area turns black and blue later, see a doctor. Even a sprained ankle can involve a small bone fracture.

5. Where appropriate, keep weight off the injured area.

6. With your doctor's permission, taking aspirin periodically over the first 48 hours may cut down inflammation.

7. Rest the injured area for as long as it takes for complete recovery. Follow your doctor's or physical therapist's advice on treatments like massage, ultrasound and deep heat.

8. Start training very slowly after injury. Use light weights, full range of motion, stretching and high repetitions to pump more blood into the area (do 20–30 reps). Heat the area first, not with a topical skin heat, but with a 10-minute hot shower or hot pack and then apply a cold after your workout. Once you injure an area, it's likely to be reinjured. If possible, avoid using heavy weights in the exercise that caused the injury.

Enough summaries, it's time to GO TO WORK!

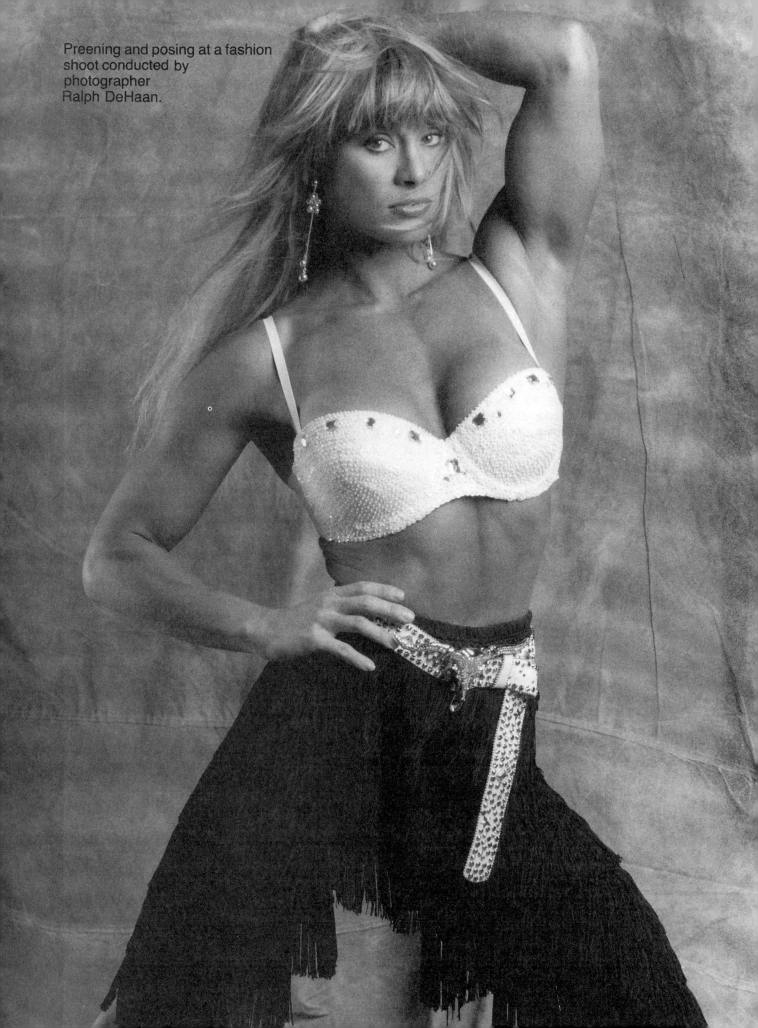

Preening and posing at a fashion shoot conducted by photographer Ralph DeHaan.

4
HOW TO DO THE BEST EXERCISES

UPPER-BODY EXERCISES

Chest

1. Push-Up

If you are weak and out of shape, start doing your push-ups on your hands and knees. Lower your upper body and face to the floor and push up with your chest and triceps muscles. As you get stronger, do your push-ups with your entire body straight (stay on your palms and the balls of your feet). Lower your body to the floor, just barely grazing the floor, and push back up to arm's length. Keep your elbows out to the sides to stress your pectoral muscles. Exhale as you push yourself up and inhale when you lower yourself down.

The chest standby—the push-up, starting position.

Elbows-out push-ups are hard but work your chest muscles well.

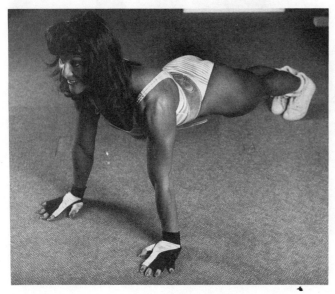

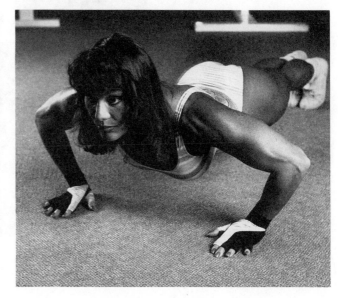

2. Incline Press

Sit back on an incline bench that has support standards. Take a pronated grip on the bar, which is slightly wider than your shoulders. Keeping your body stable, lift the barbell up and using control, slowly lower it to the high point of your chest. Inhale as you lower the bar to your chest. Without pause, push the bar back up while exhaling. For better chest development, keep your elbows out as you press the weight up. Use a spotter for this exercise.

The incline press starting position.

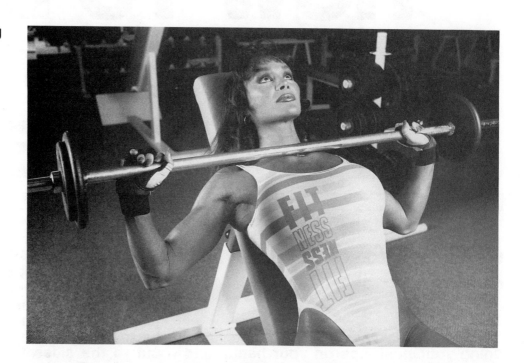

My all-time favorite pectoral exercise—the high-incline press.

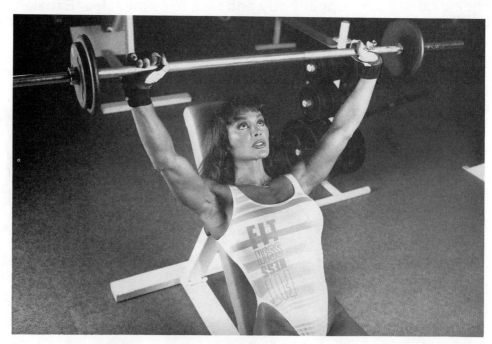

3. Incline Dumbbell Press

Position yourself on an incline bench that does not have supports, with two dumbbells at your feet, one on each side of the incline bench. Bend down and lift the dumbbells up so that you are sitting on the incline bench with the dumbbells at your shoulders, ready to push up. Push the dumbbells up together while breathing out. Keep your elbows out and your chest elevated so the emphasis is on your pectorals. Inhale and lower the dumbbells together and press them up again. Go through a full range of motion and do *not* lower the dumbbells too quickly.

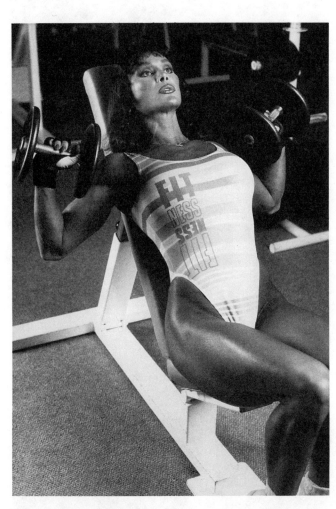

Using the dumbbells on the incline. Keep your chest held high.

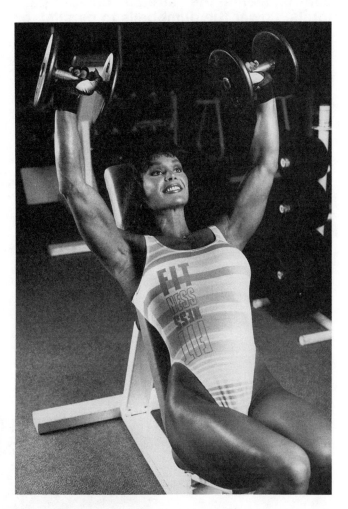

When you press dumbbells up, keep your elbows directly under them all the way to the top.

4. Incline Flye

Assume the same position on the incline bench (without supports). Press the dumbbells up to the same top position. However, hold the dumbbells with your palms facing each other. With a deep breath (and keeping your chest held high), lower both dumbbells to the sides, through a wide arc, while keeping your elbows slightly bent. Always lower the dumbbells slowly, under control, feeling the "stretch" on your pectorals. Lower the dumbbells to parallel, or just beyond parallel, with your body. Exhale and bring the dumbbells back to the starting position along the same arc through which you lowered them. The movement should resemble a bird flapping its wings. Thus the name, flye.

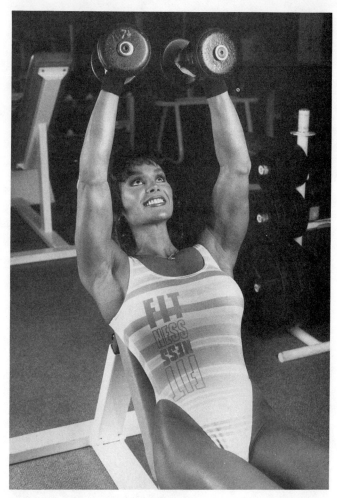

Here is the starting and finishing position for the high-incline dumbbell flyes.

Don't lower your dumbbells down too far—or too fast—and keep your elbows bent.

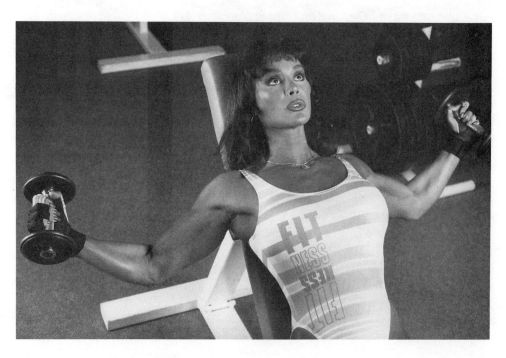

5. Bench Press

Lie on your back on a flat exercise bench with bench-pressing standards. Move under the bar until your eyes are directly under the bar. Take a pronated grip on the barbell, slightly wider than your shoulders. Lift the bar up and, under control, slowly lower it to the high point of your chest (usually your breast bone). Without pausing, push the bar back up. Do not bounce the bar off your chest. Inhale as you lower the bar and exhale as you push it up. Always keep your elbows directed out to the sides to stress your pectorals. Use a spotter for this exercise.

6. Dumbbell Bench Press

Use the exact same position as for the bench press with barbell. Pick up two dumbbells and lie back on the bench with the dumbbells at your chest/shoulder junction. Push the dumbbells up together. Breathe out as you push them up and inhale as you lower them back to the sides of your chest. Like the barbell press, keep your elbows directed out to the sides for maximum pectoral stress. Don't drop the dumbbells when you are finished. Two spotters should take them or you should lower them from your chest to your hips as you sit up and then put them on the floor.

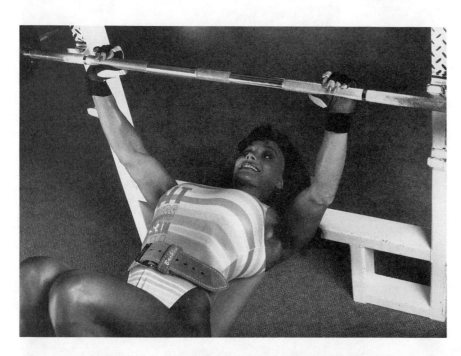

It's important to keep a stable position when you do your bench presses.

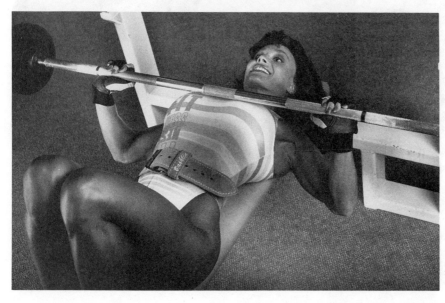

Benching with your feet up on the bench makes the lift harder, but you don't have very good stability.

7. Flat-Bench Flye

Assume the same position you would if you were going to press the dumbbells overhead. Hold the dumbbells with your palms facing each other. Take a deep breath, then lower both dumbbells to the sides while keeping your elbows slightly bent. Bring them down slowly and under control, making sure you feel a good stretch in your pectoral muscles. Exhale and bring the dumbbells back up to the starting position along the exact same arc through which you lowered them.

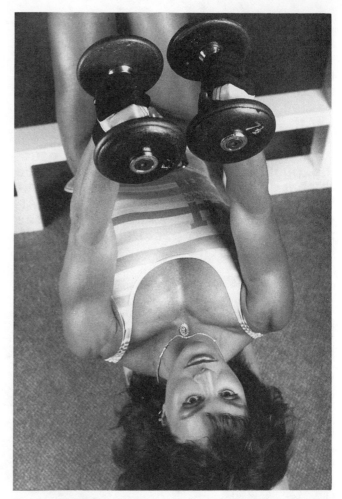

From up above, this is what the start of dumbbell flyes looks like.

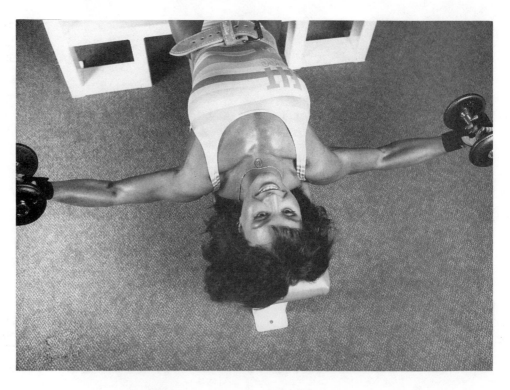

With all your flyes, don't go down too far or too fast, especially on the flat bench.

8. Dumbbell Pull-Over

Hold a dumbbell with both hands so that your palms are more or less flat against the underside of the top plates of the dumbbell. Lie back perpendicular to a flat bench so that only your shoulders are in contact with the edge of the bench (your shoulder blades should just be off the end of the bench). Your feet should be set about shoulder-width apart. Hold your head steady with your chin up. Start with the dumbbell straight over your chest and then lower it back until you get a good stretch. Keep your elbows slightly bent. Raise and lower the dumbbell through the same arc. Breathe normally and *make sure* the collars are set tight on the dumbbell. If they aren't, your face could be in danger!

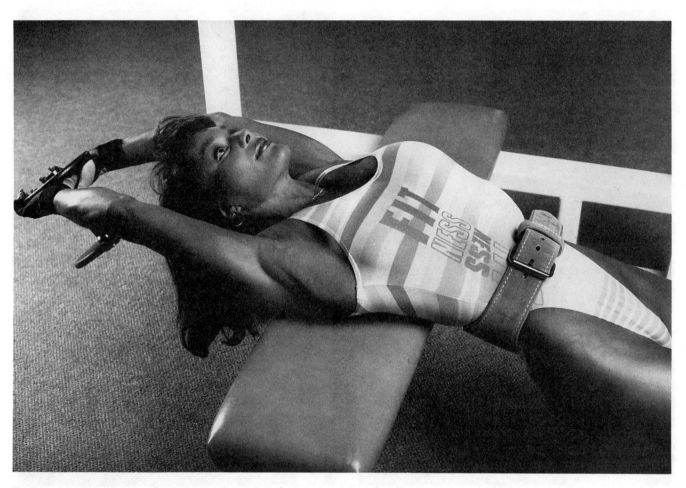

Pull-overs are the perfect tie-in exercise for your upper body.

9. Dip

Support yourself at arm's length on free parallel bars (wall-anchored or self-standing bars). Lower yourself to just beyond parallel, where the angle between your lower and upper arm is about 90 degrees. Push yourself up with your chest, arm and shoulder muscles. Breathe normally through the motion. Don't go into an extremely deep dip position unless you have very good flexibility in your chest and shoulders and only after warming up! Do *not* attach extra weights to your body for your dips.

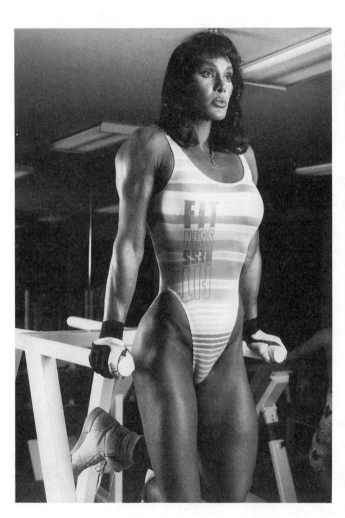

I'm psyched and ready to start my dips.

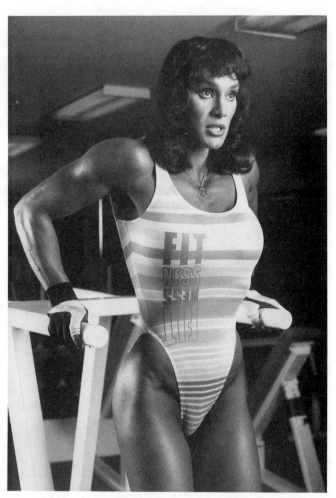

Dips are great for your deltoids, pectorals and triceps, but they ain't easy.

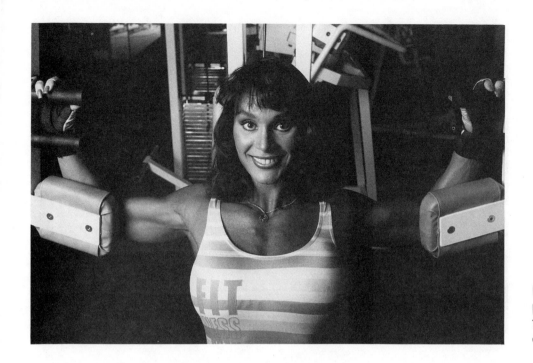

Here is the full-stretch position on the machine flye. Don't go back too far or too fast!

10. Machine Flye

Sit on the machine bench with the pads anchored against the insides of your arms at your elbow level (some machines require that you hold on to two handles, rather than use arm pads). Bring your inner forearms, at the elbows, together in front of your body. Squeeze for a second and very slowly go back to the starting position. Adjust the seat for a comfortable stretch on your pectorals. Breathe normally. You can also do machine flyes one arm at a time.

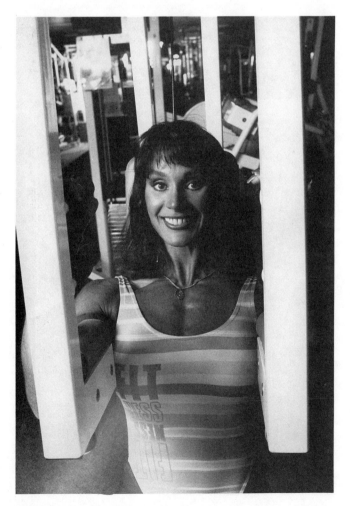

With machine flyes, bring your elbows together slowly without cheating.

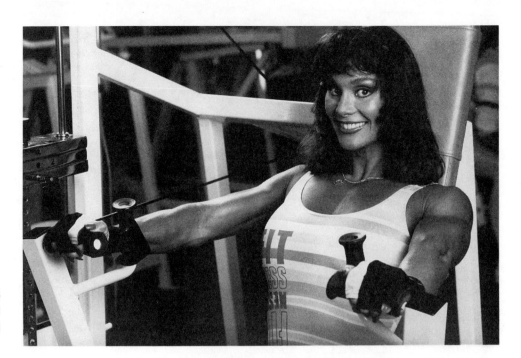

Machine bench presses are good. Here is both the starting and finishing position.

11. Machine Bench Press

The machine bench press will probably be vertical, where you push two handles out away from your body. Adjust the seat so the two handles are directly at your chest/ shoulder junction. Press the handles out to arm's length. Without pause, bring the handles back slowly and press them out together again. Breathe normally. Make sure you experiment with the seat height until you have it in the best position.

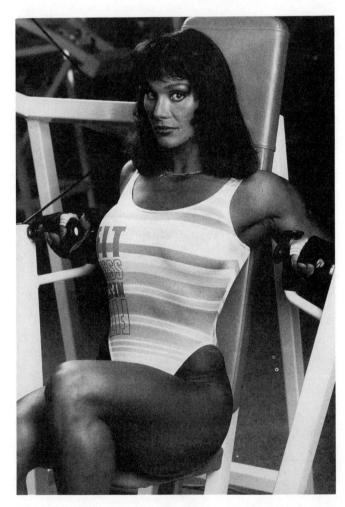

The machine bench press mid-position. You should be getting a full stretch on your pectorals.

58

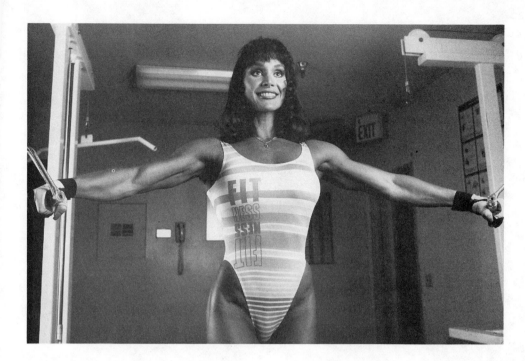

Cable crossovers work your lats, triceps and pectorals.

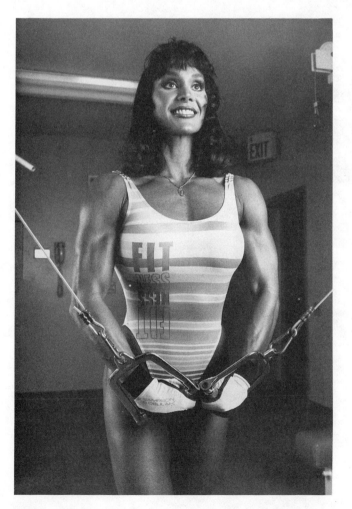

In this position you work your pectorals isometrically. Squeeze.

12. Cable Crossover

While centered between two cable stands, grasp the two handles and pull them across, slightly down and in front of the center of your body. Keeping your body in the same position, slowly resist the handles going back to the starting position. Breathe normally. As you release the handles back, make sure you get a good stretch; and don't overstretch your chest muscles at the start as this is a vulnerable position.

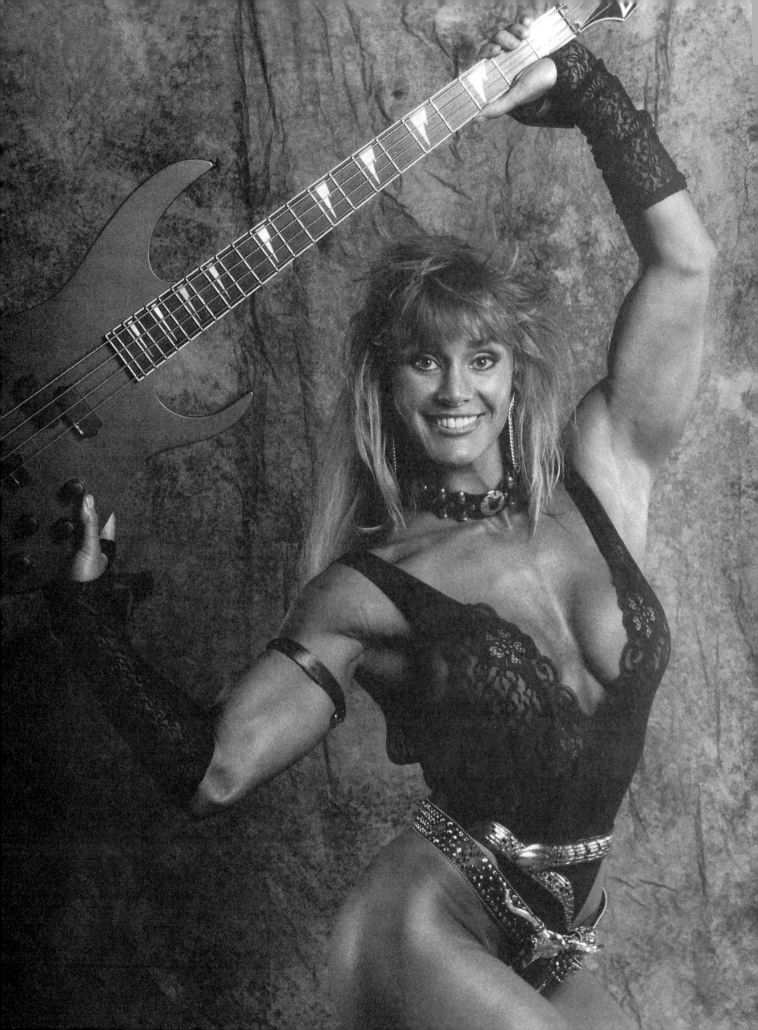

Shoulders

1. Behind-the-Neck Press

Stand or sit on the end of a bench with a bar across your trapezius muscles behind your neck. Using a shoulder-width grip, press the bar overhead to arm's length. Breathe out as you press up and inhale as you slowly lower the bar back to your shoulders. Don't rest the bar on the back of your trapezius between reps. As you press, keep the bar close to the back of your head and plant your feet to maintain solid body position. Wear a weight-lifting belt to stabilize your lower back. This exercise torques your shoulder joints somewhat, so if you have a sore shoulder(s), it may not be the exercise for you and it would be wiser to use dumbbells.

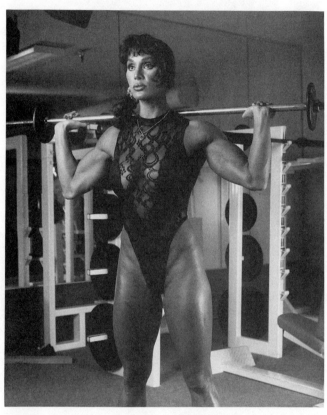

Behind-the-neck presses are a good toning movement, but can be hard on your shoulder joints.

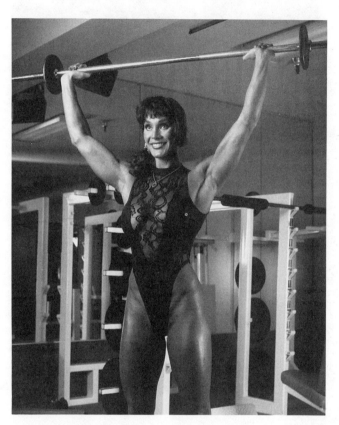

With any press, finish slowly and always under full control.

With shoulders like Cory's, if you can't play the guitar, you can at least do some behind-the-neck presses with it!

2. Dumbbell Press

In a standing or seated position, hold a dumbbell at each of your shoulders. Press one dumbbell overhead while keeping the other at your shoulder. Breathe out as you push the dumbbell up. Lower the dumbbell back down while breathing in. Now press up the other dumbbell, using the same pattern. You can press both dumbbells up together (as shown), but you have better stability when you alternate presses. For better stability, sit on a preacher curl bench so that your lower and middle back are supported.

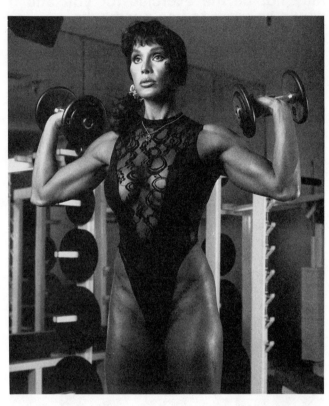

The best exercise for building shoulder strength is the press!

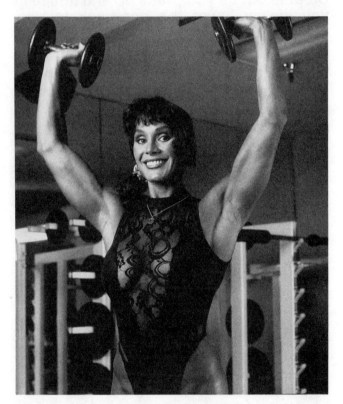

When I finish a press, I still have some bend in my elbows to keep maximum tension on my muscles.

3. Barbell Press

In this exercise, you use the same motion as the behind-the-neck press except that you lower the bar to the front of your upper chest. With front barbell presses, you go through a greater range of motion. Don't arch your back, lean backward or hold your breath. Breathe out while pushing the bar up. Wear a weight-lifting belt for support. I suggest that you use a grip about equal to the width of your shoulders.

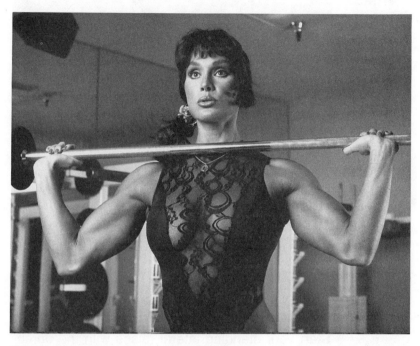

Pressing in front of your body involves more motion and requires more skill.

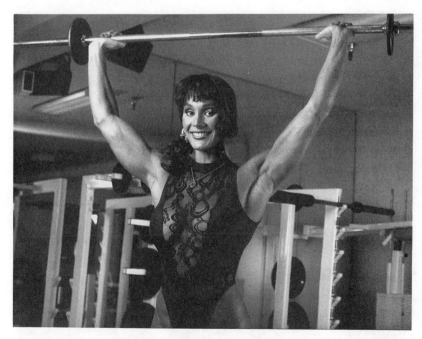

The finishing position on all your presses is always the same. Do it right.

4. Lateral Raise

You can do lateral raises either standing or sitting. Hold one dumbbell in each hand in front of your body, each against your thighs. Lean slightly forward and raise both dumbbells together to a level even with the top of your head. As you raise the dumbbells, keep both elbows and wrists slightly flexed and never let your wrists get higher than your elbows. Lateral raises are a shaping/pumping exercise. Don't cheat and try to use too much weight.

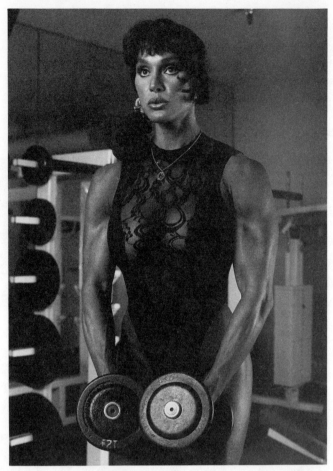

Start your standing lateral raises with the dumbbells in front of your thighs.

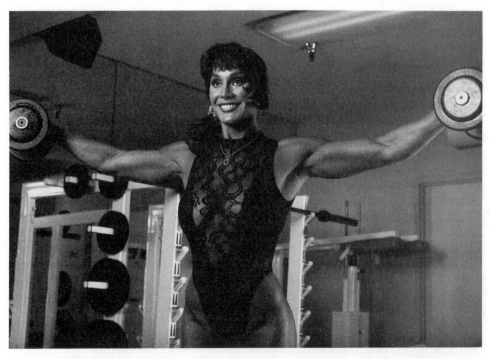

At the finish of your laterals, the dumbbells should be even with your ears.

5. Front Dumbbell Raise

Hold one dumbbell in each hand resting against the fronts of your thighs. With a slight elbow bend, raise one dumbbell up to just beyond shoulder height and return it slowly to starting position. Alternate each dumbbell. Do not lean forward and use your lower back to swing the dumbbells up. Breathe normally, exhaling when you raise each dumbbell up. You can raise both dumbbells together or do the exercise with a barbell. With a barbell or both dumbbells together, you place more strain on your lower back.

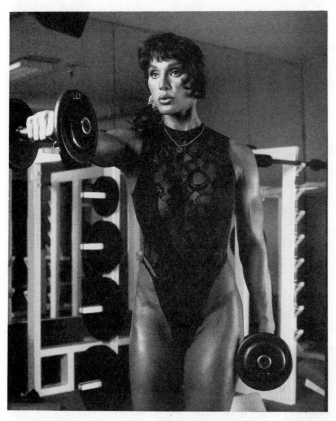

Front raises are primo for your anterior deltoids.

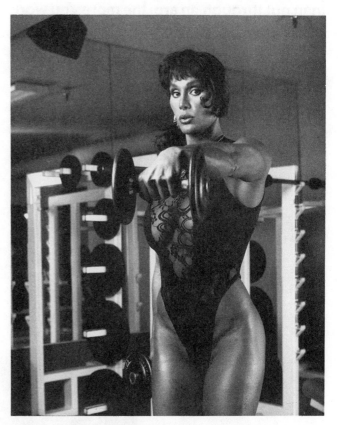

I keep my wrists flexed when I do front raises to place more stress directly on my deltoids.

6. Rear Raise (Bent-Over Raise)

Bend over with your knees slightly bent and your back close to parallel with the floor. Pick up a dumbbell in each hand and raise them out to the sides at the same time until they are slightly higher than your shoulders. Lower and repeat. Don't try to keep your arms straight. Instead, bend your elbows slightly. The more you bend your elbows and pull up and back rather than out through an arc, the more you work your inner, upper back muscles instead of your posterior deltoids. Since you're bent over and compressing your chest, make sure you don't hold your breath. If this exercise bothers your lower back, you can lie on a special bench and do the same movement. This will take your lower back out as the weak link. In any case, wear a weight-lifting belt.

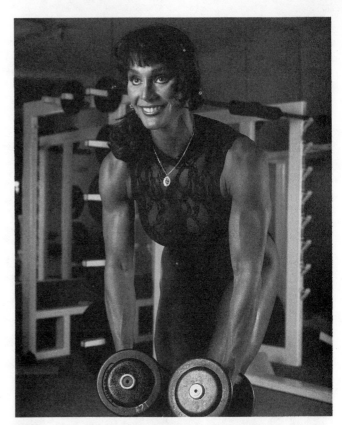

Bent-over laterals are the toughest deltoid exercise.

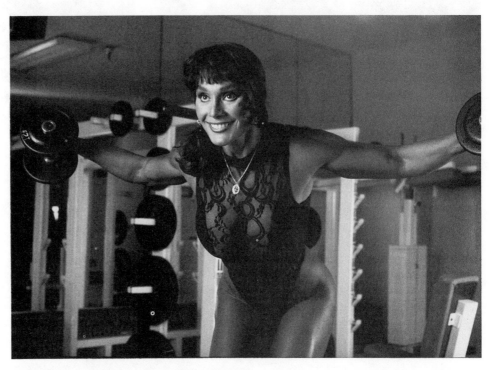

With bent laterals, I recommend light weights so you stress your rear delts and not your upper-back muscles.

66

7. Cable Lateral Raise

With cable lateral raises, you are required to exercise one hand at a time. The exercise is much the same as using a dumbbell for lateral raises, but with constant tension through the full range of motion. You can start by holding the cable handle either in front of or behind your thigh. With your elbow slightly bent, raise the handle up to just beyond shoulder level. As with any form of lateral raise, always keep your elbow higher than your wrist. Don't swing the handle up or lower it too quickly. Instead, go slowly up and down to isolate your middle deltoid fibers. This is a **technique** exercise.

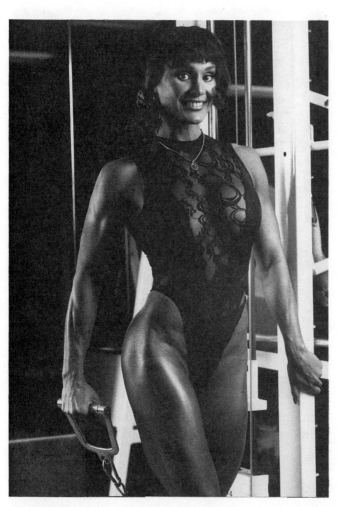

I'm smiling, but cable laterals aren't easy. Do them strictly!

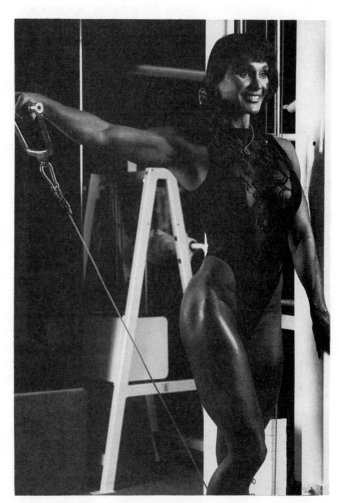

Go no higher because if you do, you emphasize your trapezius instead of your middle deltoids.

8. Shrug

Stand holding a barbell in front of your thighs at arm's length. Use a shoulder-width pronated grip. Very simply, lift your shoulders up toward your ears. Don't bend your elbows because that's cheating by using your arm flexors. You should pull your shoulders and bar straight up and hold at the top for 1–2 seconds. You can also pull your shoulders back slightly, but elevation is your prime movement. Do not bend forward and shrug the bar up with body heave. Once again, don't hold your breath.

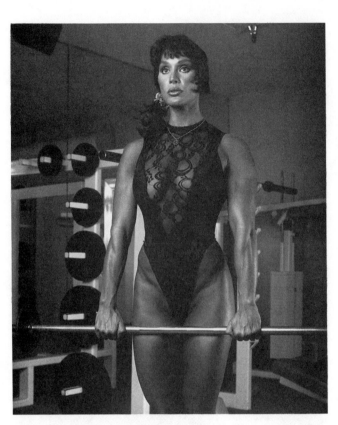

Starting out for shrugs.

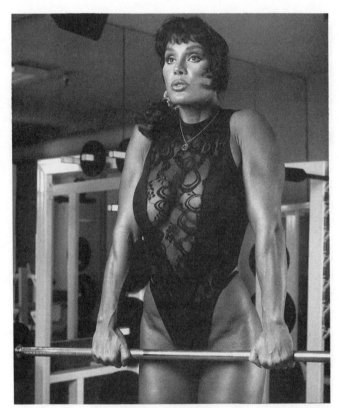

Shrugging with your elbows turned out, wrists flexed and thumbs over the bar activates your traps.

Arms

1. Barbell Curl

Stand and hold a barbell across the front of your thighs. Use either a straight or EZ-curl bar. Use a supinated grip about as wide as your shoulders (or slightly less). With your elbows in and close to your sides, slowly curl the bar up toward your neck. Don't heave the bar up with body motion or lift your shoulders or move your elbows backward too far as you do your reps. Breathe out as you lower the barbell.

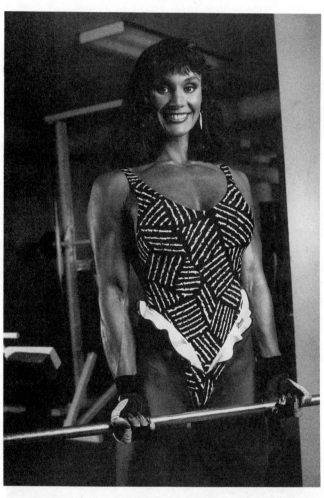

This might be the most popular weight-training exercise in existence, the barbell curl.

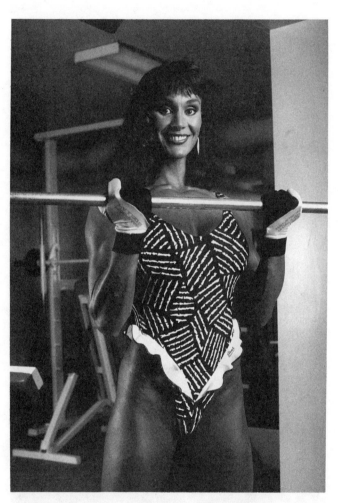

As I finish my barbell curls, I squeeze my biceps for a super-contraction at the top.

2. Dumbbell Curl

With this exercise, you can sit or stand. You can use more weight if you stand. Hold a dumbbell in each hand with a supinated grip. Staying upright, keep one dumbbell at your side and slowly curl the other up to your shoulder. Slowly lower the dumbbell back down and curl the opposite one up only after your other arm is all the way back down. Don't worry about breathing here—just breathe as naturally as possible. If you do dumbbell curls with your palms up, the emphasis is on your biceps muscles. With palms down, you work your brachioradialis and forearm extensors. In midposition, your brachialis receives most of the stress.

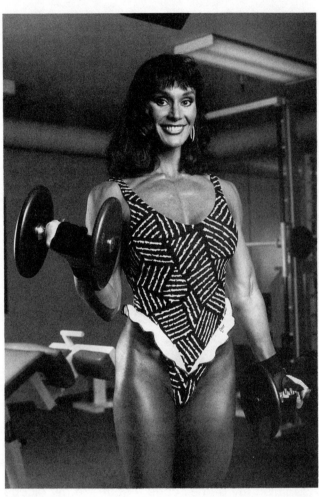

Dumbbell curls are probably my favorite biceps exercise.

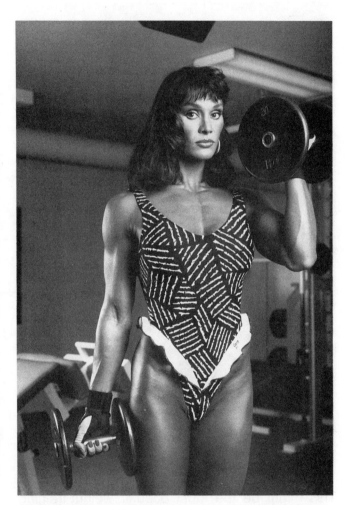

What goes up must come down. I like to alternate my dumbbell curls.

3. Scott Curl (Preacher Curl)

This exercise requires a special angled bench resembling a preacher's pulpit. Position yourself over this inclined bench so that your arms are nearly vertical over the flat part of the bench. Using either dumbbells or a barbell, and keeping your upper arms flat against the bench, slowly curl the weight up to your shoulders. It's critical to lower the bar or dumbbells *very* slowly and be extra careful at the end of the range of motion. If you lower the weight too quickly you might suffer a hyperextension elbow injury.

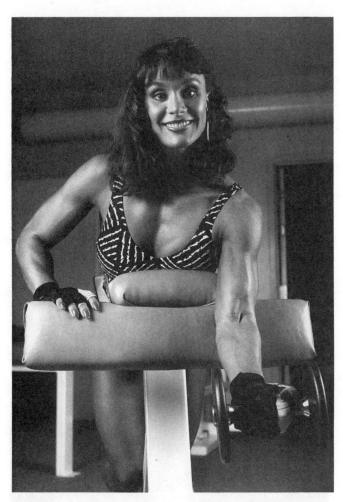

The start of the scott curl, a good exercise for your brachialis muscle.

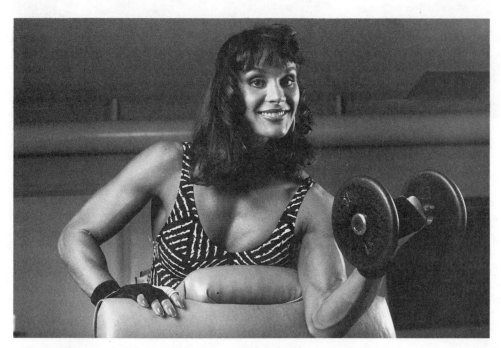

In the scott curl, don't lower the weight too far or too fast.

4. Concentration Curl

Sit on a flat bench holding a dumbbell with your extended arm bridged against the inside of your leg. Keeping your upper arm stationary, slowly curl the dumbbell up to your shoulder. When you do your curl, your opposite hand will support your lower back if you place it against your opposite thigh. Once again, it's important to lower the weight slowly to avoid potential hyperextension injury.

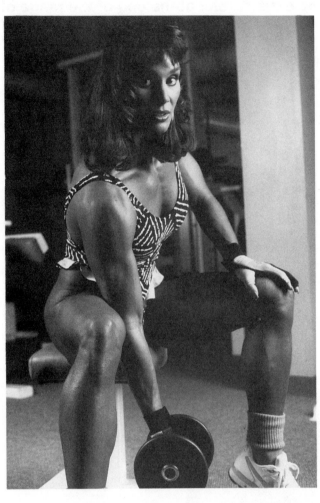

Concentration curls isolate your biceps. They're also easy on your lower back.

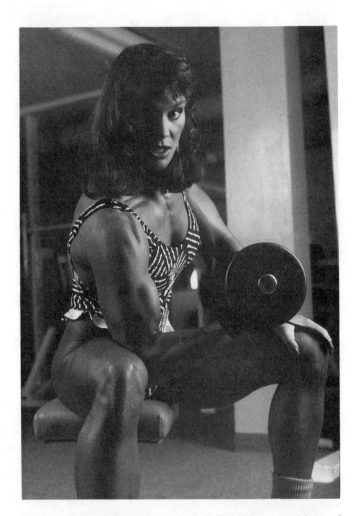

Notice that as I approach the finishing position of the concentration curl, my body position has not changed.

5. Tricep Push-Down

Stand facing a lat machine weight stack. Grab the bar with a comfortable overhead grip. Keeping your elbows in toward your sides, push the bar down through extension of your forearms until your arms are straight. Lean slightly into the weight as you push down. Slowly lower the weight back to the starting position and repeat. It's important that on each repetition you let the handle come all the way back to a full starting position. This is an isolation exercise, so concentrate on style rather than weight.

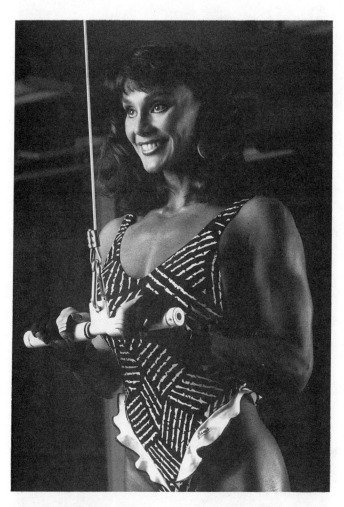

Here is the correct starting position for your tricep push-downs.

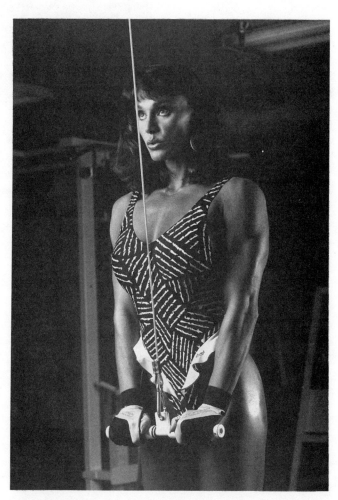

With push-downs, it's important to keep the handle close to your body through the full range of motion.

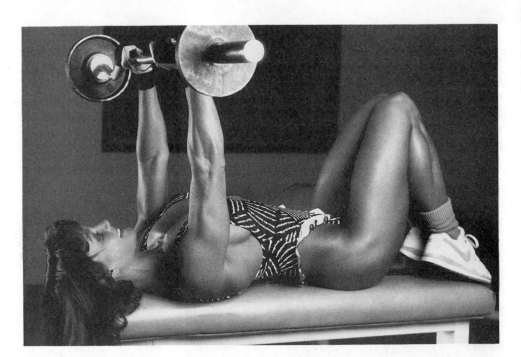

The lying tricep extension works the belly of the three-headed tricep muscle. Here's the start and finish.

6. Tricep Extension

You can do extensions standing, sitting or lying down. If lying, position yourself on a bench holding an EZ-curl or regular bar using a narrow, pronated grip. Push the bar up to arm's length. With your elbows stationary, lower the bar down behind your head all the way past the end of the bench. After lowering the bar as far back as you can, straighten your elbows, returning the bar to the upright starting position. Don't hold your breath, instead, breathe normally.

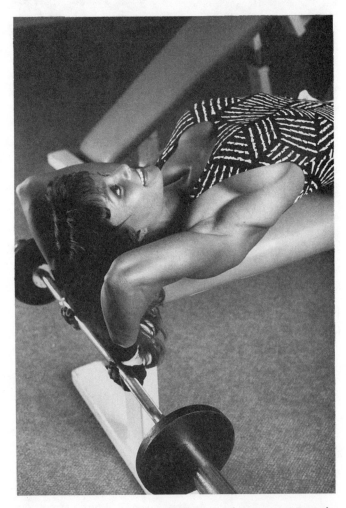

I go below my head to place my triceps on stretch for a better, more powerful contraction.

7. Tricep Kickback

Supporting yourself with your hand and knee on a flat bench, hold a dumbbell with your other hand and bend at your elbow. Keeping your elbow fixed, move your lower arm back into extension until your arm is straight. Try not to move any part of your arm except your forearm with your only movement at your elbow joint. Slowly lower the dumbbell back to the bent-elbow position. Do all repetitions with one arm before switching to the other arm.

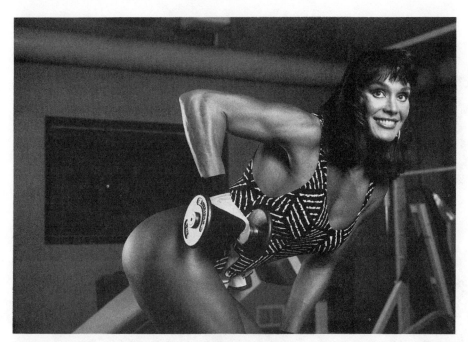

Kickbacks work your triceps without abnormal stress on your elbow joints.

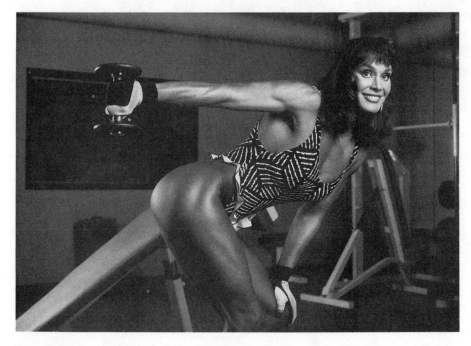

The finishing position of the kickback. Full range of motion is always preferred.

8. Reverse Curl

Hold on to a barbell with your arms extended so that the bar is against the front of your thighs. Use a pronated grip. Keeping your elbows stationary, slowly reverse-curl the bar up to your shoulders. Lower the bar slowly and repeat. Do not use excess body motion, lift your shoulders or swing the bar up. Most people have 30 percent less strength in the reverse curl as compared to the regular curl.

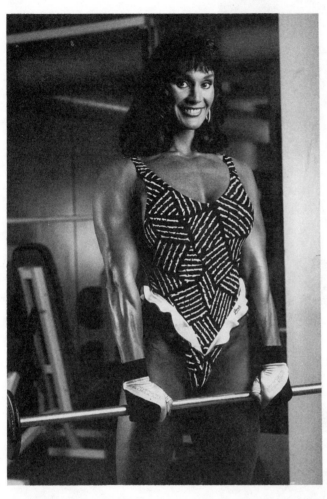

Don't forget your forearms! Here I'm starting my reverse curls.

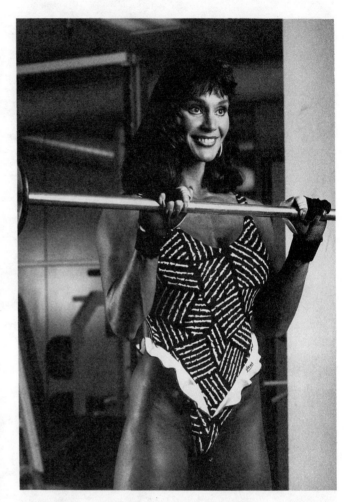

It's critical with reverse curls to keep your elbows against your sides. Use your forearm muscles, not your back muscles!

9. Regular Wrist Curl

Sit at the end of a flat bench with your forearms resting on your thighs so that your wrists hang over your knees with your palms up. Using a narrow grip on a straight bar, or using dumbbells, flex your wrists up through a full range of motion. Very slowly lower the bar or dumbbells back to the starting position and repeat. Forearms respond best to high reps. Using heavy weights for low reps may strain your wrists rather than build your muscles!

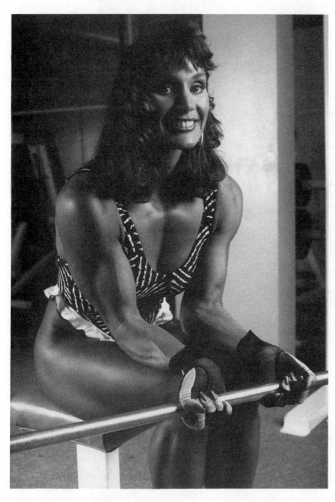

Problems with tennis elbow and weak wrists? Do the regular wrist curl for high repetitions. Here's the starting position.

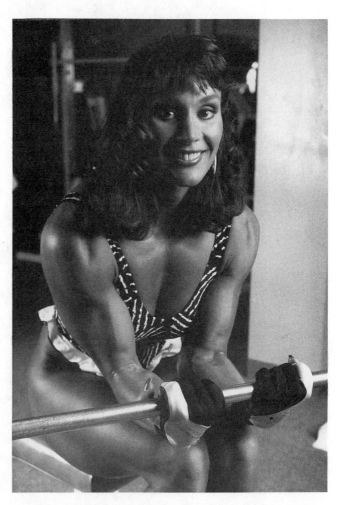

When finishing your wrist curls, don't lift your forearms off your thighs.

10. Reverse Wrist Curl

Use the exact same technique as the reg- ular wrist curl but with a pronated grip. You'll be much weaker in this position so use less weight.

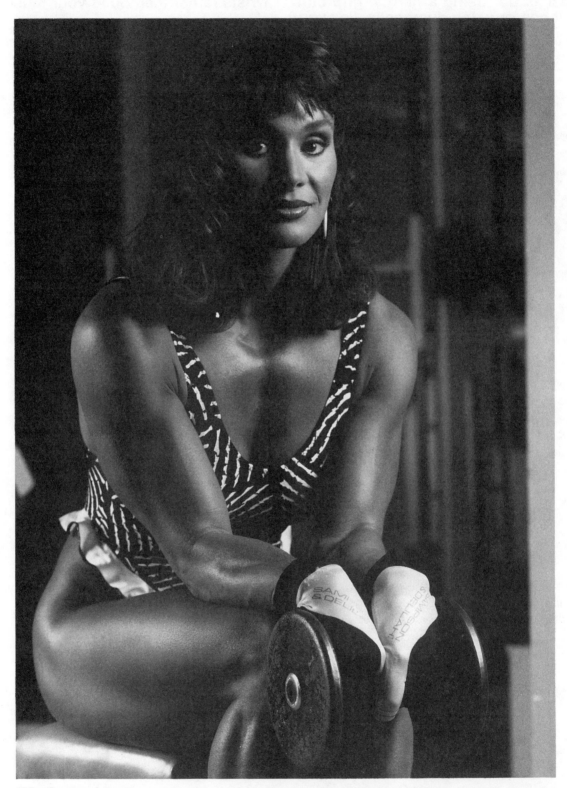

What's good for the goose is good for the gander. If you do regular wrist curls, you must do reverse wrist curls to keep your muscles in balance.

11. Pull-Up

With pull-ups, technically, if you use a palms-up (supinated) grip, you'll be doing a chin-up, with the emphasis on your biceps muscles. If you use a palms-away (pronated) grip, you'll be doing a pull-up with the emphasis on your forearm and upper-back muscles. In any event, pull yourself up high enough so that your chin is at the level of the bar and don't use unnecessary body action or swing. Concentrate on the pulling action of your arms.

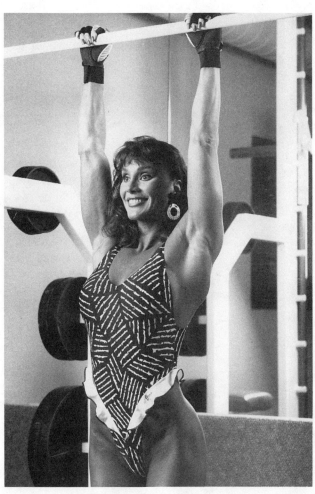

I'm not just hanging around doing nothing. This is the start of a hard set of close-grip pull-ups.

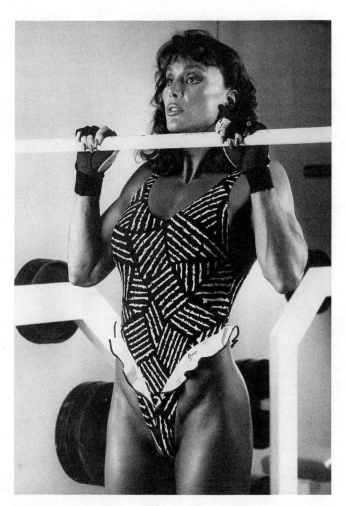

Pull-ups are really tough. Use a spotter if you need help finishing each repetition.

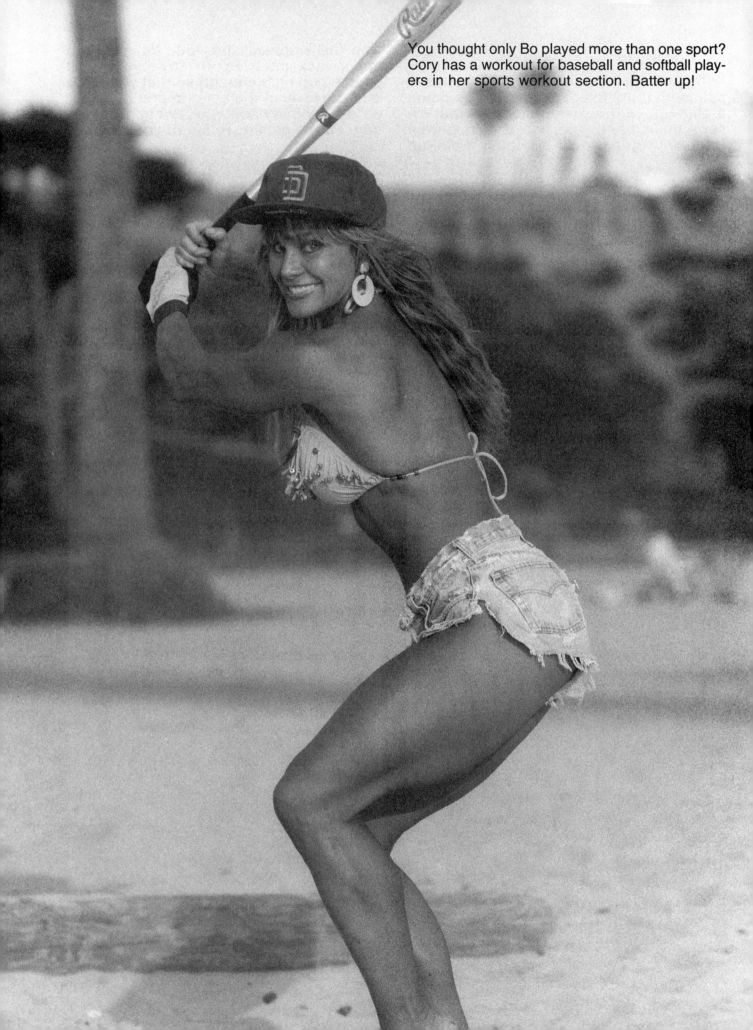

You thought only Bo played more than one sport? Cory has a workout for baseball and softball players in her sports workout section. Batter up!

Back

1. Wide-Grip Pull-Up

This is the exact same movement as the regular pull-up except you use a wide grip, at least 2–3 inches wider than the width of your shoulders. Try to maintain a slight arch in your lower back, keep your chest held high and actually try to pull your chest toward the bar. This will ensure that you get a good muscle action from your lats and upper-back muscles. It's a difficult exercise and you should enlist a spotter to help you with your last repetitions. Hand straps will also help your grip.

2. Lat Pull-Down to the Rear

Start in a seated position facing the lat machine. The tops of your thighs should be anchored under the upper seat. Grasp the overhead bar with a comfortable grip (the wider the grip, the harder it is to pull the weights down and the more isolation there is on your back muscles because your arms are weaker in this position) and pull the bar down until it grazes the back of your neck/shoulder junction. Don't pull the bar down fast. Pull slowly. Keep your chest elevated and bring your elbows way back and down. Exhale as you pull the weight down and inhale as you resist the weight going back.

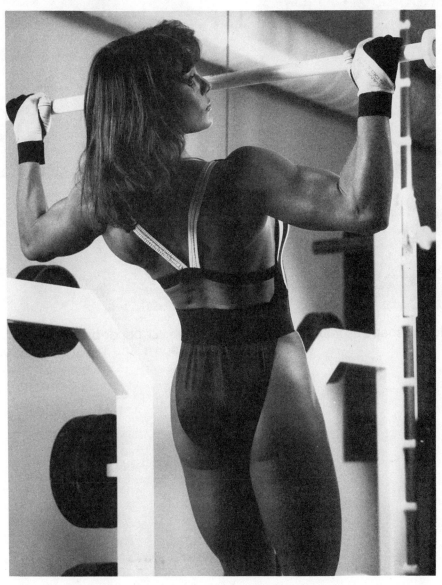

Wide-grip pull-ups are really tough, but boy, do they improve your upper-body shape and endurance.

3. Lat Pull-Down to the Front

Use the same position as in the rear pull-down. Pull the bar down to the high point of your chest while keeping your lower back slightly arched. With all back exercises, bring your elbows down and back behind your body to isolate your lats. Don't "round-over" and cheat by using reverse action of your pectoral muscles. Use the same grip as you do with pull-downs to the rear, but vary it from workout to workout. Use a V-handle if you want greater emphasis on your biceps.

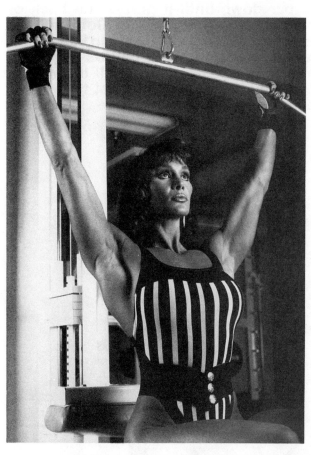

Lat machine pull-downs shape up your upper back quickly!

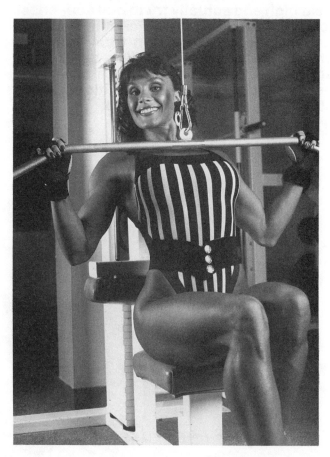

As with all upper-back exercises, bring your elbows down and back behind your body as you finish.

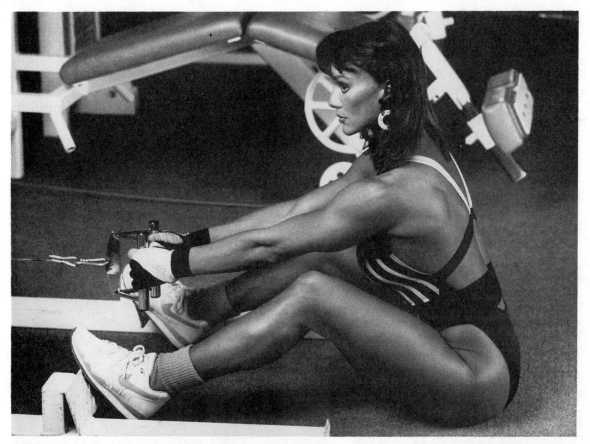

When you stretch on your long pulley return, stretch your lats not your lower back! Be careful!

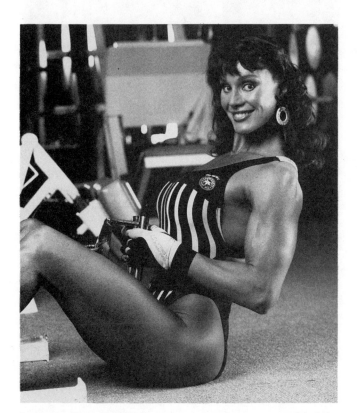

Long pulley rows fully pump your inner, upper back muscles.

4. Long Pulley Row

Sit with your feet blocked against the long pulley support bar with a slight bend in your knees. Lean forward and grasp the exercise handle (you can use either a V-handle or a straight bar). From a moderately stretched position, pull the handle in toward your stomach, bringing your elbows way back at the end of the motion. Don't swing the weights up and don't overstretch your lower back at the forward part of the exercise; this could lead to injury. Exhale as you pull the weight up and breathe in upon the return.

5. Bent-Over Row

Bend over your barbell, keep your back just slightly above parallel to the floor and maintain a 10–20-degree bend in your knees. This will remove stress from your lower back. Hold the bar with a pronated grip equal to your shoulder width and pull the bar up so that it touches your navel region. Concentrate on your upper back muscles and draw your elbows way back and up. Don't yank the weight up or hold your breath. If this exercise bothers your lower back switch to one-arm dumbbell rows.

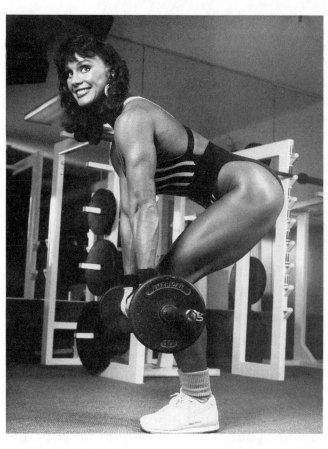

Here's the mid-position of the flat-back deadlift. Never round your back over.

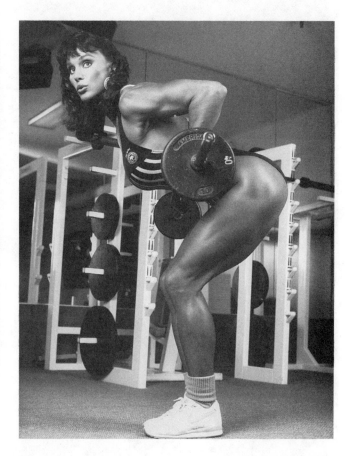

Notice as I finish a bent-over row that I maintain the same flat back position as I do in the deadlift.

6. One-Arm Dumbbell Row

Start with one hand and knee propped up on a bench while holding a dumbbell in your opposite hand. Keeping your back flat with your other knee slightly bent, pull the dumbbell up from a fully stretched position to your shoulder/chest junction. Hold the dumbbell at the top for a second if you can and then lower it slowly. Again, concentrate on bringing your elbow up and back with your lats at the end of the rep. Inhale as you pull the weight up and exhale as you resist the dumbbell coming down.

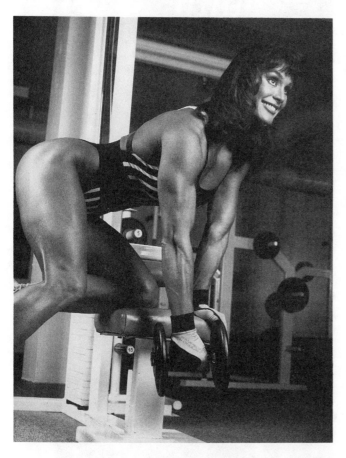

The one-arm row gives you freedom and support while you isolate your latissimus muscles.

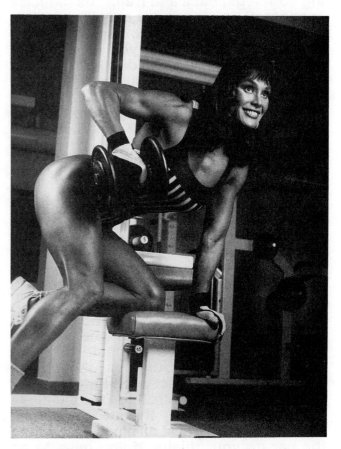

Bring your elbow behind your body during the finish of the one-arm row.

7. Power Clean

This is a difficult exercise and several sessions must be spent learning technique. Keeping your back as flat as possible, bend your knees and hips, lean down and grasp a barbell with a pronated shoulder-width grip and pull the bar to your shoulders. The pull to your shoulders should be an accelerated motion, slow-to-fast, utilizing your legs, back and trapezius muscles in concert. Your arms are only "hooks" on to the bar to impart force generated from your legs and back. As you rack the bar on your chest, you should only bend your knees a few degrees. If you drop way down to fix the bar to your shoulders, you're not doing a power clean. Don't try to use too much weight. Concentrate on speed, form and power.

8. Shrug

The shrug can be considered both a back and shoulder exercise. See the description of the shrug under shoulder exercises.

9. Flat-Back Deadlifts

Stand with your shins just grazing the barbell. Bend down naturally and hold the bar with one hand forward and one hand reversed or both hands pronated if this is comfortable. With your hips, thighs and lower back, stand erect while keeping your back as flat as possible. Keep the bar close to your shins during the lift. Your arms should stay straight at all times. Don't drag the bar up your thighs. If you have to do this, you're using too much weight. It's very important not to use too much weight or to round your back over at the start because you can injure yourself.

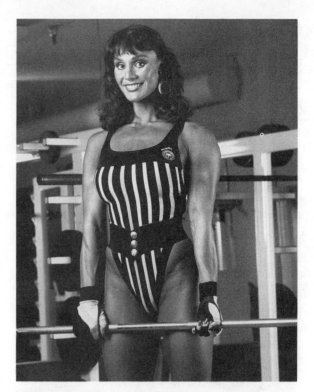

Here's the finishing position for the flat-back deadlift. Notice I have one hand pronated, one supinated.

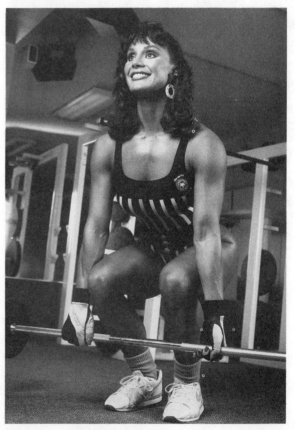

When you deadlift, use your thighs, hips, butt and back in unison.

10. Hyperextension

Lie off the end of a special bench face down. Your feet and lower leg area should be anchored. You should bend your upper body over a supported pad so you can raise up and down in comfort and freedom. Lower your upper body all the way down and then raise it up until your upper body is just beyond parallel (do not overextend). Slowly lower yourself back down and repeat. Breathe normally. Do higher reps in this exercise. Hyperextensions bother some people. If it bothers you, do the same movement while lying prone on the floor instead.

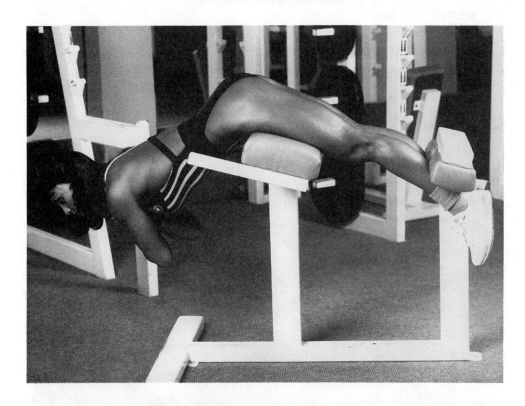

This is my recommended starting position for the hyperextension exercise.

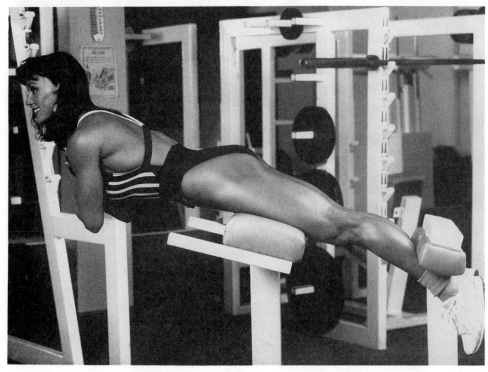

Don't go up any higher than just slightly beyond parallel when you do hypers.

Abdominals

1. Side Sit-Up

Lie on your side with your knees together and slightly bent. Put your upper hand against your head and try to sit up sideways, concentrating on flexing your oblique abdominal muscles at the end of the movement. (You can't come up too high—this is a concentrated short movement.) Do your side sit-ups slowly and do an equal number of repetitions for each side without any rest between sets. To make side sit-ups harder, do them off the end of a bench with a partner anchoring your legs. You can work your obliques even harder in this position by adding a twist as you come up.

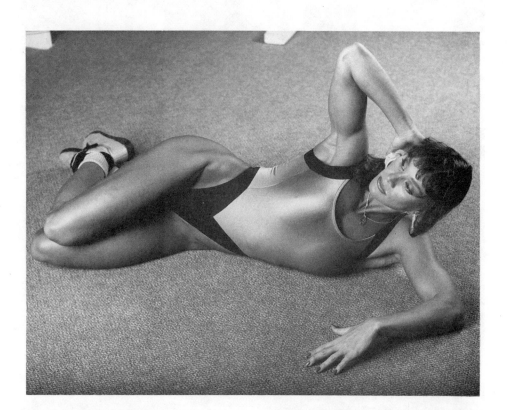

Side sit-ups are very effective for toning your obliques.

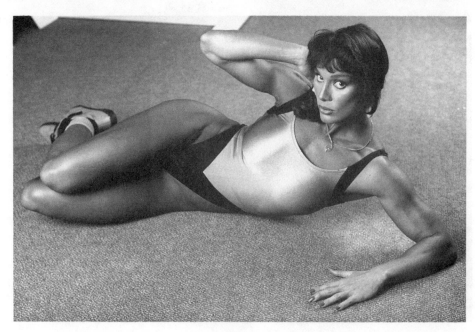

With side sit-ups, concentration and style are most important.

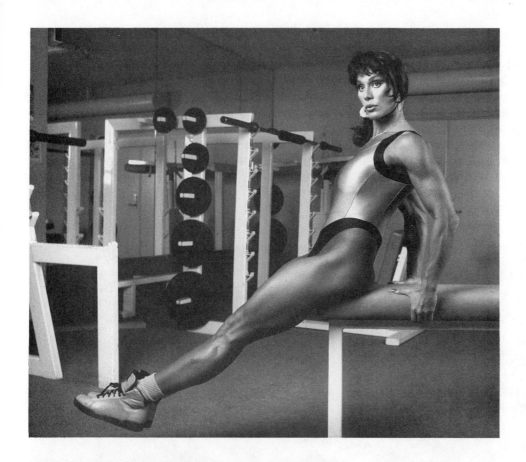

To do straight-leg raises, sit at the end of a high bench. Be careful—sit on a sturdy bench.

2. Leg Raise

Sit on the end of a bench with your upper body inclined backward about 10 degrees. Tighten your abdominals and slowly raise your legs off the floor until your feet are as high as your head. If you have weak hip flexors and abdominals, start with one leg at a time. Keep your legs straight or you will only tire your hip flexors (the more your knees bend, the more the emphasis switches to your hip flexors). Don't lower your legs like a ton of bricks. Instead, lower them slowly, under total control. This works your abdominals eccentrically. Inhale while lowering your legs, exhale while lifting them up.

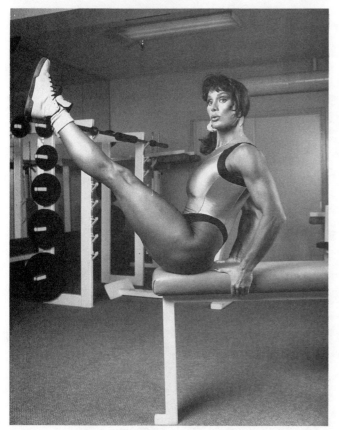

Straight-leg raises condition your upper-thigh, hip and abdominal muscles.

3. Lean-Back Twist

Anchor yourself on a sit-up board that has a foot attachment, or on a flat bench where you can hold on to some piece of the equipment with your feet. Lean back with a 45-degree angle between your upper body and the floor. Twist slowly to one side and super-contract your oblique muscles at the end of the range of motion. Hold for a second and then twist all the way to the other side and do the same contraction.

Keep a constant tension on all of your abdominals, but don't twist too fast. If you hold on to a weight plate or dumbbell or a bar behind your neck, the exercise is much harder. With extra weights, you add a force at the end of the range of motion, so your twist must be even *slower* than before. Exhale at the end of the ranges of motion to each side while you squeeze your obliques. This will make the exercise more effective.

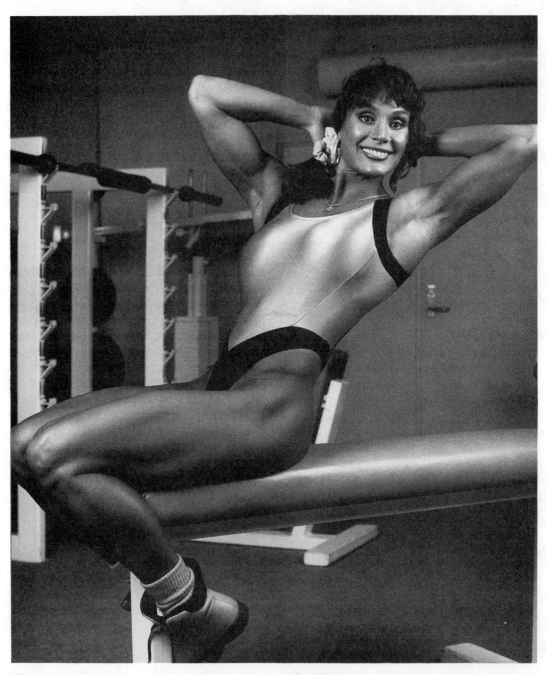

Twisting sit-ups do nothing unless you lean back as you do them, move slowly and squeeze your muscles at the end of your twists.

4. Crunch

Lie on the floor on your back. Bend your knees up to 90 degrees over a support chair or bench or hold them up using muscle action. Push your lower back into the floor (the pelvic tilt position which activates your abdominals), and slowly curl your upper body toward your legs. Curl up high enough so that your shoulder blades clear the floor by about 1–2 inches. Exhale as you crunch, concentrating on a super-contraction at the end of the crunch.

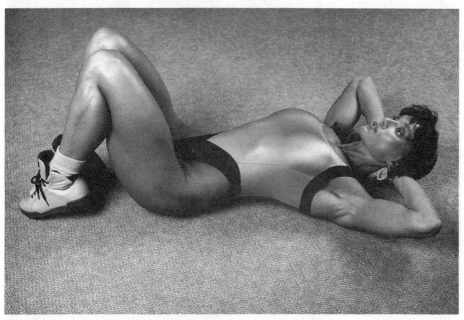

Here is my relaxed starting position for the Cory crunch, your basic abdominal exercise.

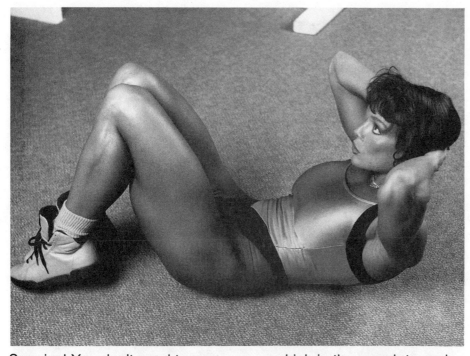

Surprise! You don't need to come up very high in the crunch to work your rectus abdominals.

5. Advanced Leg Raise

This is a difficult exercise, but very effective. Lie on your back on the floor or on a bench. Keeping your shoulder blades and mid-back fixed, curl your lower body up as high as you can, going up onto your shoulders. From this position, slowly lower your pelvis and legs to a parallel position, making sure you hold the muscle tension. Without relaxing, pull your torso and legs back up again. This is one repetition. Breathe normally and concentrate on stressing the lower section of your abdominals.

Believe it or not, this is the starting position of a very advanced reverse leg raise. Lower your legs slowly.

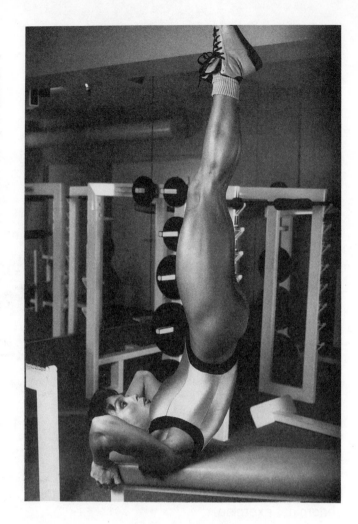

I'm halfway down in an advanced reverse leg raise and it's getting hard.

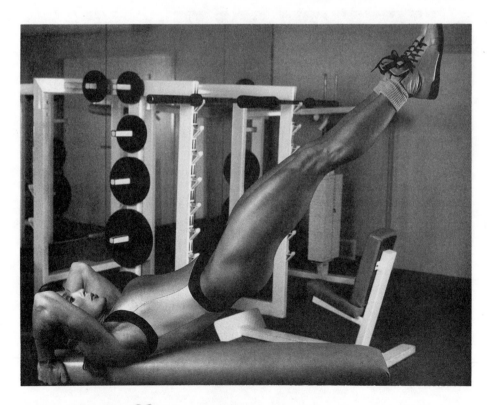

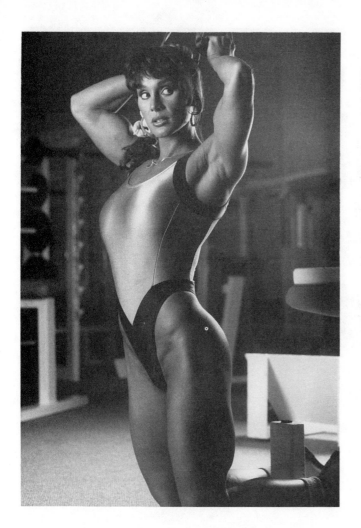

6. Lat Machine Crunch

Position yourself on your knees facing the lat machine. Give yourself enough room so that you can bend forward all the way without touching any part of the machine. Grab the handle or bar, holding it right by the top of your head. Slowly bend forward bringing your face toward your knees. Flex your abdominals strongly at the bottom position. Blow your air out as you curl down into the bottom. Inhale as you go slowly back to the starting position. To activate your obliques, pull down in a sideways direction.

Here is the starting position in the lat machine pull-down crunch.

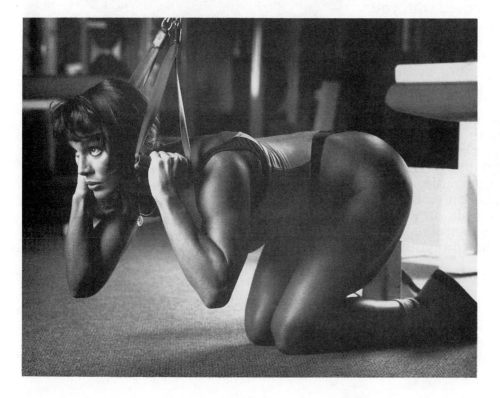

Keep your arms fixed when you do pull-downs. Just flex your abds, not your triceps!

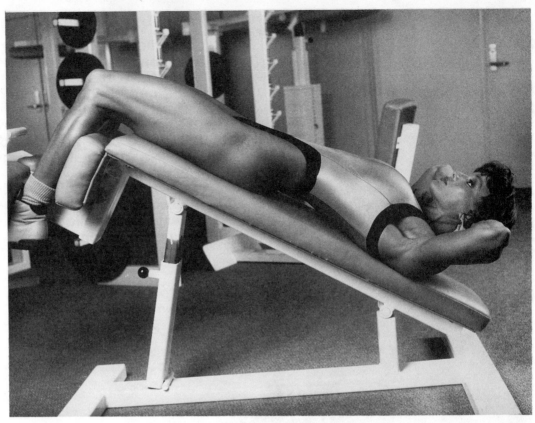

Sit-ups on a steep angle are an advanced exercise.

7. Incline Sit-Up

Sit on an adjustable sit-up board with your feet anchored (you should select a bench where you can bend your knees). Tighten your abdominal muscles, flex your chin to your chest and slowly (without swinging at the start) curl yourself up. Then, lower your body slowly back to the starting position. It's important to go very slowly. It's not absolutely necessary to go through a full range of motion, especially if the exercise bothers your lower back. This exercise does pull on your hip flexor muscles, which, in turn, pull on your lower spine. Therefore, some people may experience discomfort from this exercise. If this happens, drop the exercise from your program.

Remember, anchoring your feet automatically stresses your hip flexors and this can cause back strain in some people.

94

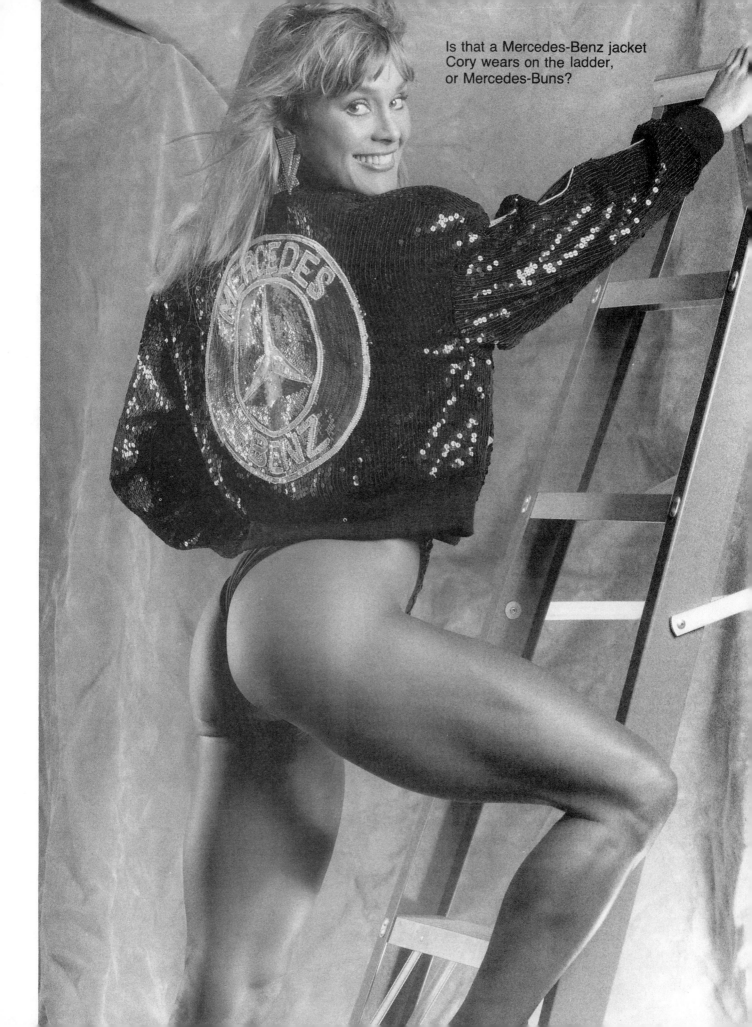

Is that a Mercedes-Benz jacket
Cory wears on the ladder,
or Mercedes-Buns?

LOWER-BODY EXERCISES

Hips

1. Side-Lying Hip Abduction

Lie on your side and raise your top leg straight up. If you keep your leg straight the exercise is harder. Bending your knee improves your leverage and is easier. Don't rest your upper leg at the bottom between reps. This exercise isolates your gluteus medius, although with your leg straight you also work your tensor muscle on the side of your thigh. Do repetitions for both legs. If you raise your leg up and forward, you're substituting with your front thigh muscles. If your leg drifts backward, you're substituting with your glutes and hamstrings. As you get stronger, add ankle weights or do this with the standing pulley machine!

Side-lying leg raises for your hip abductors look easy, but believe me, they're not.

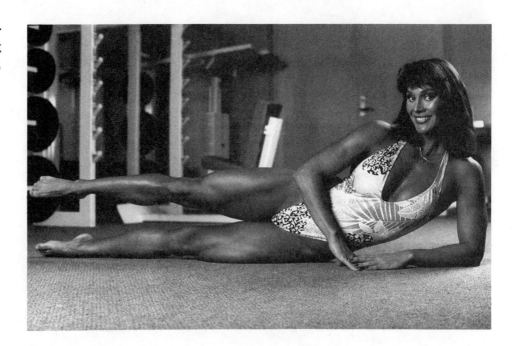

Abductor leg raises work your gluteus medius and tensor thigh muscles. They'll shape, slim and tone you fast.

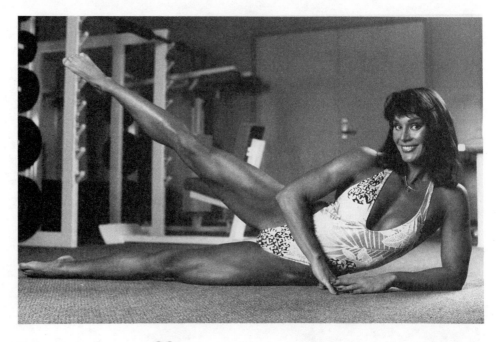

96

2. Hip Flexion

You can do this exercise sitting or standing. Keep your leg straight and raise it in front of your body. If you bend your leg, all the tension goes to your psoas muscles. With your leg straight, you work both your hip psoas and rectus femoris of your quadriceps group. Don't rest between reps. Once you're stronger, you can wear ankle weights or do the exercise seated with weights over your lower thighs.

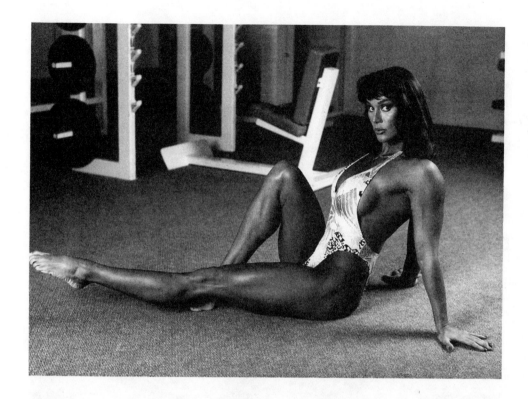

I'm not relaxing, but getting ready to do a set of hip flexor leg raises.

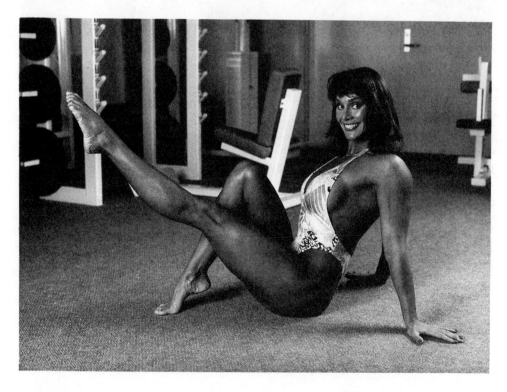

This is as high as you need to go in the hip flexor raise. Try for 20 reps!

3. Hip Adduction

Start in the same position as you do in side-lying hip abduction. This time hold your upper leg up and bring your lower leg up to touch your upper leg. It's tough! You might only be able to do a couple reps to start with, but you'll gain strength quickly.

To make it easier, you can bend your bottom leg and bring it up while bent. This gives you better leverage and strength. You can also do adduction using the pulley machine. Stand sideways to the pulley machine and hook a cuff around your knee or ankle and pull your inner leg away from the machine.

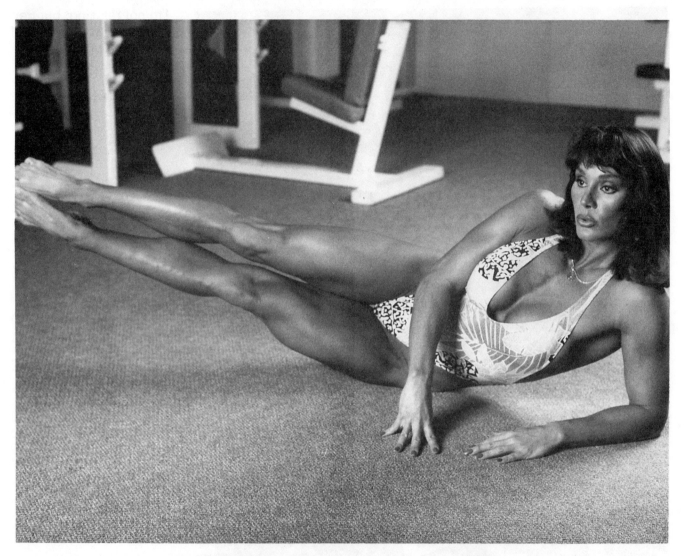

Don't neglect your inner-thigh (adductor) muscles. Lift your top leg up and bring your bottom leg up to touch it. Sound easy? Don't count on it. See if you can do 10 good ones.

4. Hip Extension

Start out on all fours (hands and knees). Raise your leg up and back. If you raise your leg bent, the emphasis is on your gluteus maximus. With your leg straight, you work your hamstrings more. Don't try to lift your leg up too high because you have to arch your lower back to accomplish this and this may invite injury. **To make the exercise harder, use ankle weights. You can also face a pulley and, with the cuff around your ankle, move your leg backward into extension.**

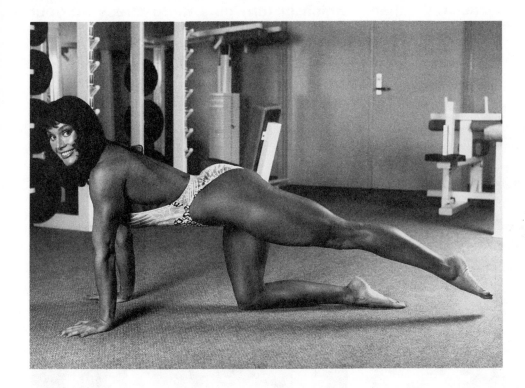

Hip-extension straight-leg raises are wonderful for toning up weak hamstrings.

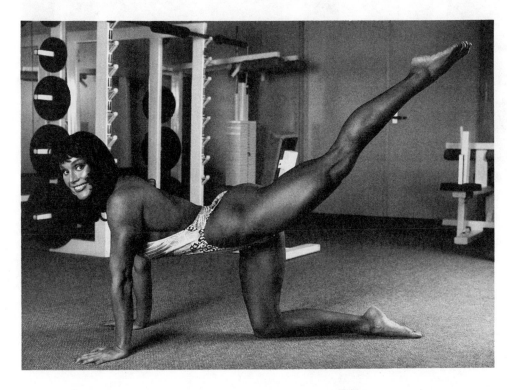

When hip extensions get easy, add an ankle wrap-around weight to increase your resistance or use a pulley machine with ankle cuff.

Thighs

1. Squat

Stand with a barbell across the back of your trapezius muscles. Use a grip (wide or narrow) on the bar that is most comfortable for you. Position your legs where your feet are at least shoulder-width apart, but preferably about 3–4 inches wider than your shoulders. Your feet should not point straight ahead, but instead, angle outward at a 45-degree angle. Keeping your back flat, squat down to a point where the tops of your thighs are parallel with the floor. Make sure when you go down and come up that your knees are always in the same direct line as your feet. Descend slowly and wear a weight-lifting belt. Additionally, at first use a 2–3″ block under your heels when you squat. With your heels elevated, you can keep your back more upright, which in turn puts more stress on your thighs. Learn technique with an empty bar before you start adding weights. At your option, you can also wear knee wraps.

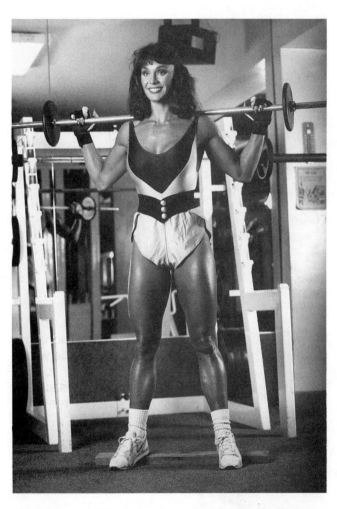

I'm getting ready to start the best exercise in weight training—the squat. I like to raise my heels.

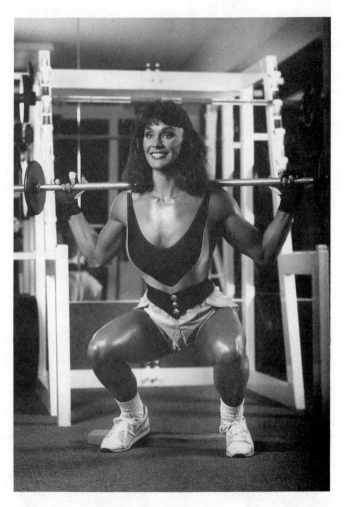

This is a good depth for the squat, thighs parallel to the floor.

2. Smith Machine Squat

Stand exactly as you would for a regular squat except your feet should be closer together and slightly in front of your body.

Smith Machines have built-in hook attachments that you guide with your hands to start and finish your repetitions. Using the Smith Machine allows you to squat up and back, further isolating your thighs!

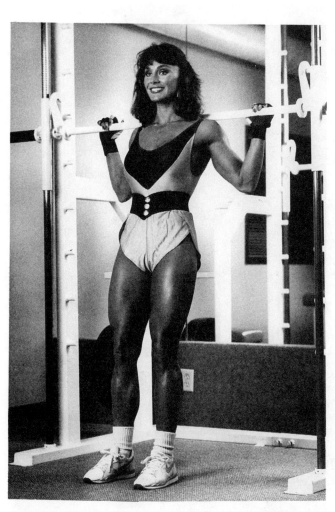

Squatting front-to-back using the Smith Machine. What a great thigh pump!

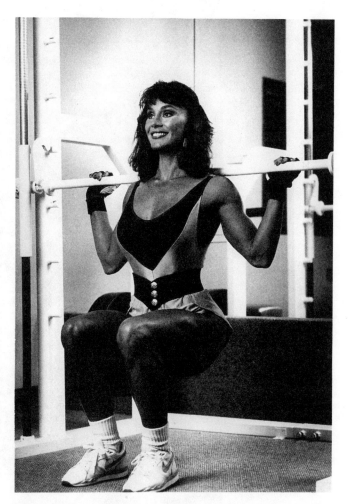

It's easy to maintain a straight-back position in the Smith Machine. That's why it's so effective.

3. Hack Squat

To do this exercise properly, use a special machine. Start in the extended top position with your shoulders underneath two pads and your hands on two special handles. Position your feet so you are comfortable for the duration of the exercise. With your feet down low and close together, you'll work more of your quadriceps. With your feet high and wide, you'll work your quads and your glutes and hamstrings, too. Release the safety catches and slowly descend into the squat position. To start with, descend only to a point where the tops of your thighs are parallel to the floor. Don't bounce, drop or relax into the bottom position. Constantly flex or tighten your thigh muscles during the exercise. When pushing yourself back up, keep your knees parallel to each other in the same direction (pointing out ever so slightly).

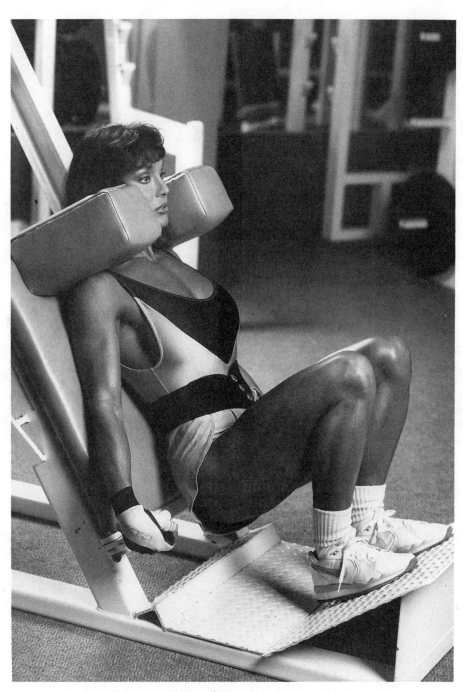

This is midway through a hack squat.

4. Leg Press

Sit in a special machine. Position yourself comfortably, with the seat adjusted for efficient leg excursion. Place your feet on the board following the same principles as with the hack squat: low and close together for quads, high and wide apart for glutes and hamstrings. Release the safety catches and slowly lower the board until your legs are almost fully bent. When lowering and pressing, keep your knees in the same direction. Don't rebound out of the bottom or pause at the bottom between reps. Press the weights up smoothly. Never jerk the weight up or attempt to change your foot position while completing a repetition. When you have completed your repetitions, rehook the safety mechanisms. Exhale as you push up, inhale as you lower the weights.

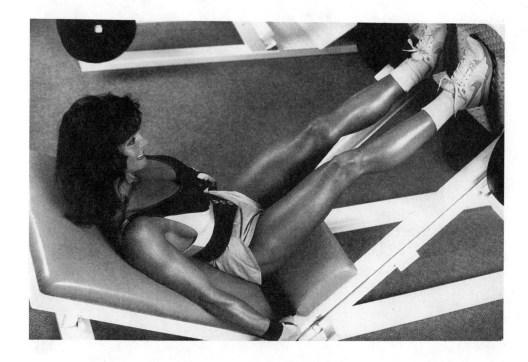

Here's the start of the leg press. Maintain a comfortable foot position.

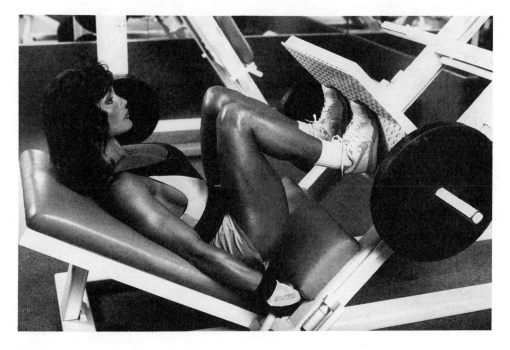

Don't cramp yourself at the bottom of your leg presses. Don't go into too much knee flexion.

5. Leg Extension

Sit on a special quad-extension machine. The backs of your knees should be flush with the lever arm of the machine and your ankles behind the foot pads. Holding on to stabilizing handles, extend your lower legs through a full 180-degree range of motion. Hold the top position for a second and then lower slowly while keeping your torso stationary.

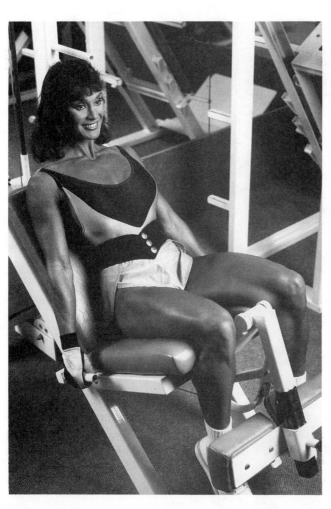

Leg extensions are numero uno for your quadriceps tone.

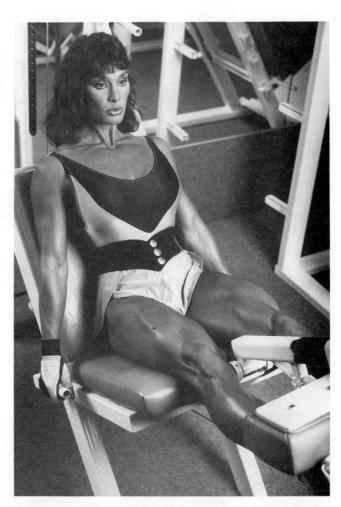

Go for a full 180-degree extension as you finish.

6. Step-Up

Like some of the other quadricep exercises, the step-up not only works your quadriceps, but also your glutes and hamstrings. To begin with, don't use any weights in this exercise. Step up onto a low bench (I recommend 6–20″) doing all your reps with one leg before switching to your other leg. At your option, you can go up on your toes to complete the step-up. The higher the bench, of course, the more difficult the exercise and the more potentially stressful to your knees and lower back. After a while, you'll be able to hold dumbbells or carry a barbell across your back when doing the step-up. However, this isn't a good exercise to pile on a lot of weight. Instead, emphasize good form.

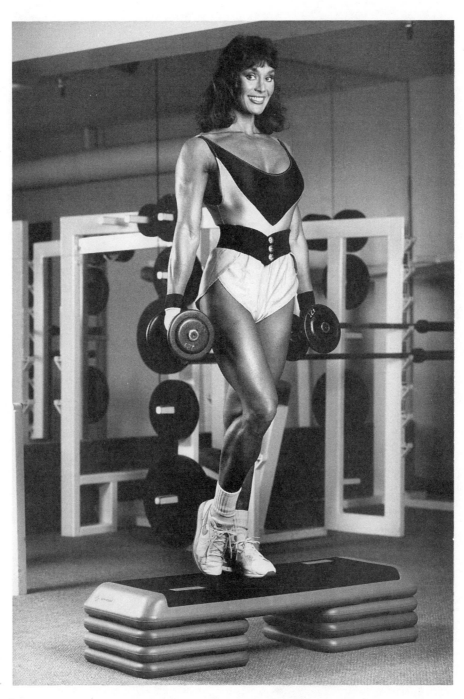

As you get into better shape, you can add weights to some of your low-impact aerobic movements, for example, the step.

7. Lunge

Start with a barbell across your back (or you can do this exercise while holding dumbbells or without weights at all). Take a comfortable step forward and slowly descend into a flexed-knee position (the angle between your thigh and lower leg should not be in excess of 90 degrees as your knee tendon receives a lot of strain in this position). Push back up to the starting position except don't go up all the way. Instead, stop about 5–10 degrees short of a fully locked-out position. This will keep constant tension on your quadriceps muscles. Do all your reps on one leg before switching to the other. You should also experiment by lunging onto a short block, which allows you to go into a deeper position without as much strain on your patellar tendon.

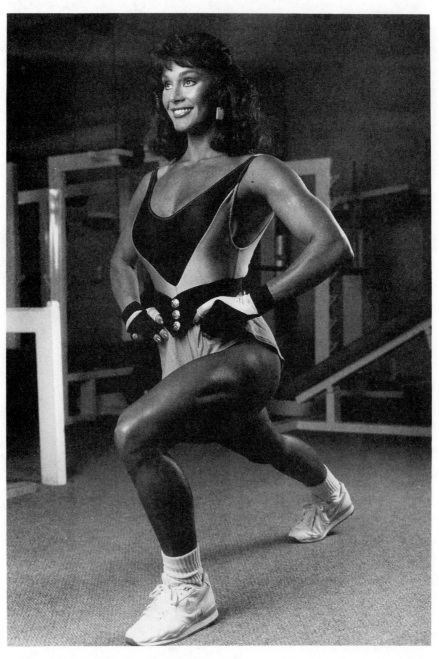

Lunges work many muscle groups, so they should be a part of your non-weight exercise program.

8. Cory Lunge

With this exercise, you maintain the same position as with the regular lunge, but instead of stepping forward, you step backward and descend into a flexed-knee position. There is less stress on your patellar tendon and you work your muscles eccentrically in the primary motion. My Cory Lunge works your glutes and upper hamstrings more than your quadriceps. The principles are the same—do all your reps on one leg first before the other, and when you come up, stop about 5–10 degrees short of lock-out to maintain constant tension.

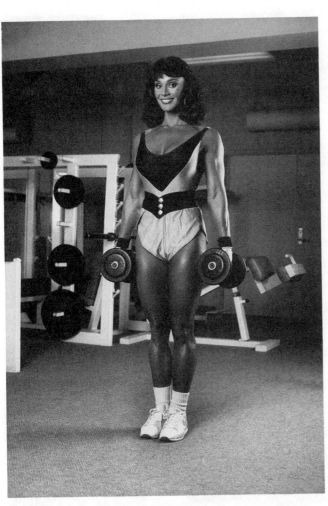

I'm getting ready to do the dumbbell lunge.

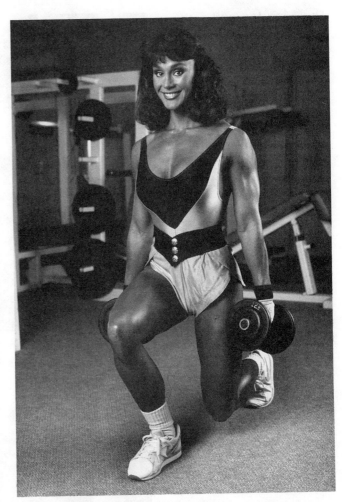

I don't want you to do a deep-knee-bend lunge. It puts too much pressure on your patellar tendon in your knees.

Hamstrings

1. Lying Leg Curl

Lie on a special machine, stomach down. Your knees and lower legs should be off the end of the bench with pads behind your ankles and lower legs. Anchor yourself with your hands so you are in a stable position. Slowly curl your lower legs up as close as possible to your upper thighs and glutes. Don't jerk the weight up or lift your rear end off the machine. Always lower the weights slowly. Exhale while lifting the weight up, inhale as you lower the weight. It is not easy to start a leg curl, so you are limited to how strong you are at the start of the exercise. In my opinion, you shouldn't try to handle a great deal of weight. Instead, concentrate on slow, good reps with tight form.

The lying leg curl works your hamstrings in its leg flexing function. Your hamstrings are also hip extensors.

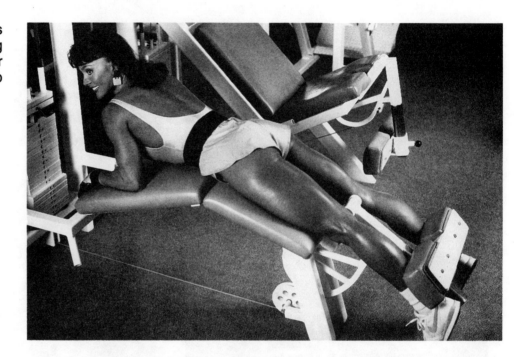

I like to do high reps (12–20) in the lying leg curl to shape up my legs.

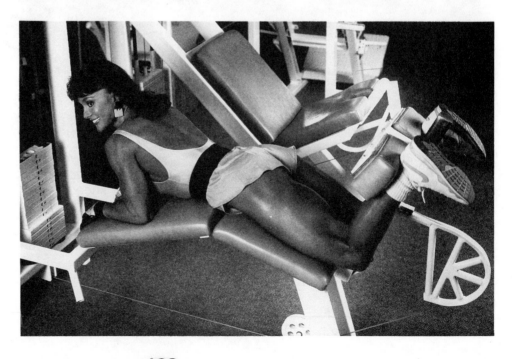

2. Standing Leg Curl

This exercise requires a special machine. With your body secure and with a pad over your heel tendon, curl your lower leg up so that your heel moves toward your upper thigh. Do all your reps on one leg before switching to your other leg. It is more difficult to get a full range of motion in your knee joint in this exercise. So, you can't use maximum weights and trying to do so places your lower back at risk.

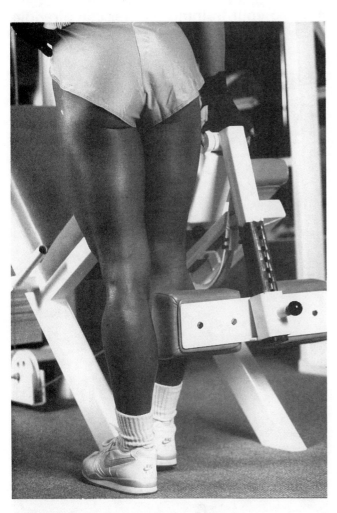

Starting out in the standing leg curl.

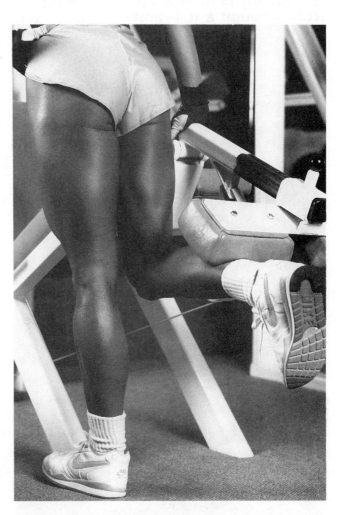

The mid-position in the standing leg curl. A great one for your hamstrings!

Calves

1. Standing Calf Raise

Stand erect on a block with the pads of a standing calf machine on your shoulders. Raise up on the balls of your feet on the foot board as much as possible and hold for a second. Slowly lower yourself so that your heels go well below the foot board. Maximum height and depth is important for growth. Keep your knees locked out, or just slightly bent, when doing your raises. Work through a full range of motion and don't try to use so much weight that you strain your lower back rather than work your calves. Wear a weight-lifting belt and breathe normally.

2. Donkey Calf Raise

Use a calf block like you do with standing calf raises. Place the balls of your feet on the block and rest your arms on a padded bench supporting your upper body at a parallel position to the floor. Squat down a bit so your training partner can straddle

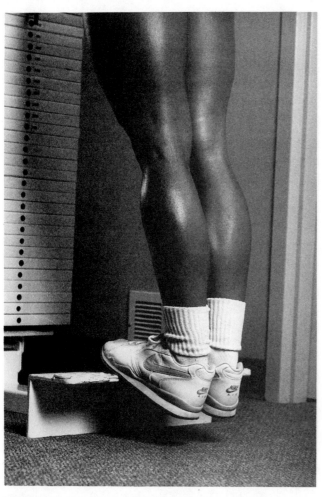

Heels way down in the standing calf raise!

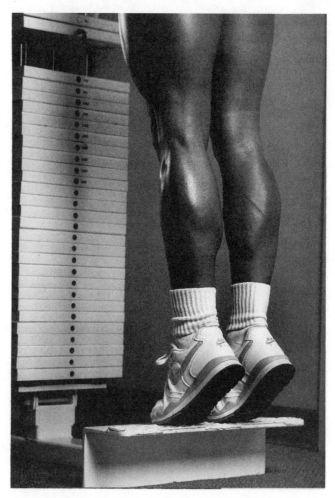

Heels way up in the standing calf raise!

110

your hips, riding low. Straighten up and proceed to do your calf raises, up and down, with your partner coming along for the ride—providing the resistance. Go through a full range of motion for maximum stretch, all the way up and hold for a second and all the way down. If you're going to use maximum weights for any of your calf exercises, do it on the donkey raise. You can attach weights around your waist with a belt if you don't have a training partner.

3. Seated Calf Raise

Sit on a special machine with the balls of your feet on a block and a special pad over your knees, across the tops of your thighs. You can use dumbbells, weight plates or your partner for resistance if you don't have access to a seated calf machine. Remove the machine's safety catches and rise up on the balls of your feet through a full range of motion. Hold for a second at the top and then lower slowly so that you get another full range of motion (and stretch) at the bottom.

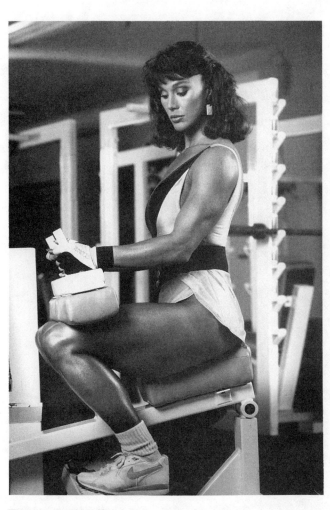

The seated calf raise is great for your soleus muscles.

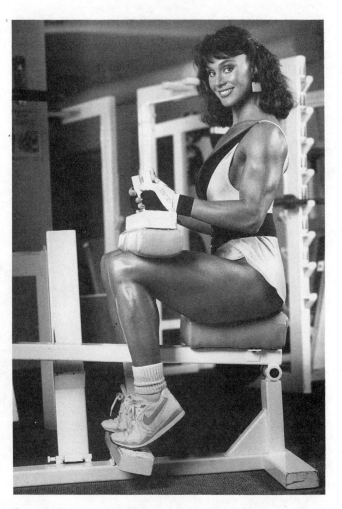

Go all the way down on your toes. Full range of motion builds muscle best.

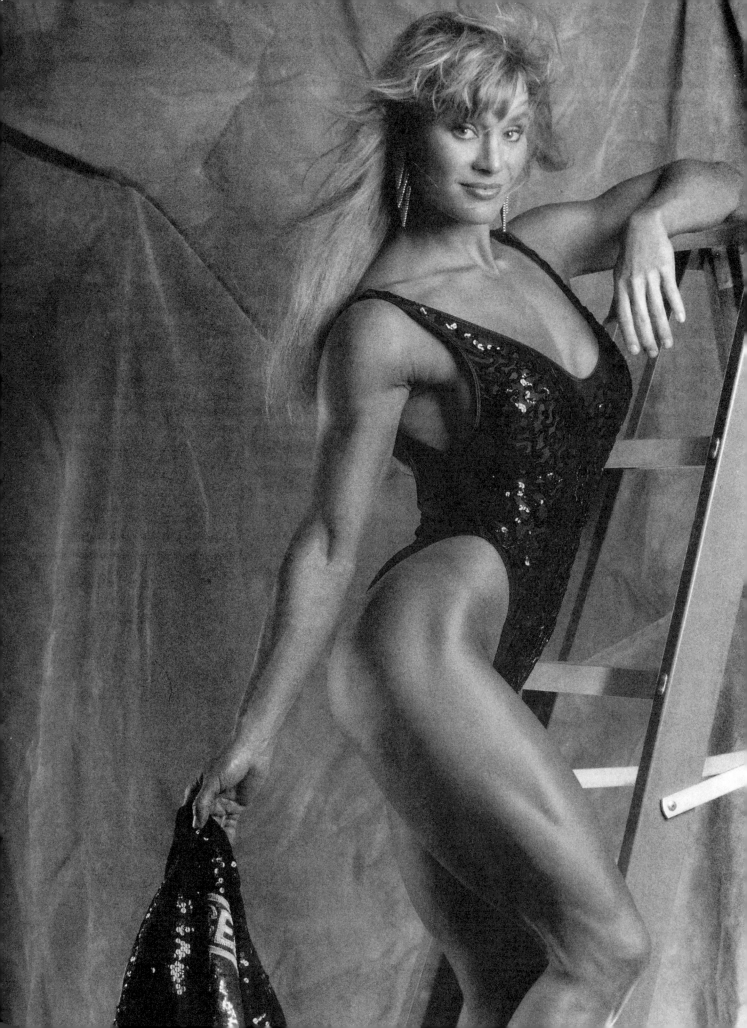

5
WORKING YOUR UPPER BODY

CHEST

Basic exercises build basic bodies. You can build your chest muscles (pectoralis major and minor) with push-ups. After a while though, you'd stop growing from push-ups, although you'd continue to gain better chest, shoulder and arm muscle endurance. You wouldn't stop getting stronger completely, but your rate of increase would slow to a crawl because you don't have any way to progressively overload your chest, shoulder and arm muscles.

No matter how many push-ups you do, unless you find a way to make them harder (like adding weight to your back), you won't get as far as you could.

One of the problems with any exercise program is boredom. Who has the motivation to just do push-ups every chest workout? With a variety of exercises you won't get bored and you will get better workouts.

Some exercises are clearly better than others. If you had only enough time and energy to do squats, lat machine pull-downs and bench presses, you could build a shapely, firm body.

Squats work your glutes, quadriceps, hamstrings, lower-back erectors and many other muscles. Pull-downs work your lats, upper-back muscles, trapezius, arms (biceps) and rear deltoids. Bench presses work your pectorals, triceps and deltoids. You can do a lot with a little.

A Lot of Chest With Little Training

Most bodybuilders do the same chest-building exercises. The bench or incline press is a starting point, but this assumes you've mastered the push-up and basic pressing technique first. You may have read somewhere that bench presses are not good for your shoulders; but you get shoulder problems from bench presses because you bench *too* heavy *too* often, not because the exercise is so bad.

Others claim that bench presses work only your shoulders and don't work your chest muscles. Bench presses, whether machine, bar or dumbbell, build your pectorals if you use a relatively wide grip (I recommend slightly wider than your shoulder width to start) and press the bar or dumbbells up with your elbows pointed out away from your body. Keep your upper

You've heard about the "ladder of intensity" in bodybuilding? Now this is what we call intense.

113

and lower arms at a 90-degree angle all the way through the exercise.

When competing, I used flat dumbbell or barbell bench presses and incline presses with the bench set at different angles. My favorite chest-shaping and building exercise is the incline dumbbell press. High-repetition chest exercises work for me in building and shaping my chest. I do sets of 10–15 reps for most of my chest exercises and I use a pyramid method a lot.

In a later chapter I will tell you how to perform all the good weight-training exercises. Study and practice them carefully. I'll list my favorite chest exercises and how I do them in my workout. In "Putting It All Together" I merge chest exercises with other body parts in your workout. Chest workouts in isolation don't help much.

When I train upper body, I train chest first. Usually, after chest, I work shoulders and upper back or arms or sometimes just chest and shoulders. I do a lot of sets and my workouts can last two hours. My workouts are advanced and intense and I don't recommend them for beginners. However, chest-training principles are the same for everybody.

My Favorite Chest Exercises

Study my chapter on how to do the best exercises and then practice them to make your best progress. The incline dumbbell press is a good shaping/building exercise because most women are too skinny around their collarbones (clavicles).

I use an adjustable bench (my favorite angle is about 45 degrees). This works your upper-chest muscles and even more when you use a high-angle bench (75 degrees, for example)!

I use a pyramid method. I start with light weights and work heavier while lowering my repetitions. Then, I lower my weights and increase my repetitions. For example, I start with 20 reps with a light weight and then gradually move up to a very heavy weight for 10–12 repetitions. Altogether, I do 5–8 sets of 10–20 repetitions of incline dumbbell presses.

The incline press, although a strong shaping exercise, is mainly a power/strength/size builder. The incline flye is a pure shaper. Sometimes I superset incline presses with incline flyes. Technique is

very important. Don't use a lot of weight for your incline flyes. If you use too much weight, you'll screw up your form, use muscles you don't want to use and rob your pectorals of the work they need. In my workout, I do 3–5 sets of 15–20 reps of flyes.

I used to do a lot of regular bench presses. In fact, at one time I could do 200 pounds for 10 repetitions. I don't train as heavily now since I'm not competing anymore. To maintain tone, strength and shape, I do machine bench presses. This exercise works your pecs without abnormal shoulder stress. Four sets of 12–15 repetitions works for me.

Also known as a pec-deck, I like to alternate machine flyes with machine presses. The machine flye is a bit different than the dumbbell flye. With machine flyes, there is always constant tension on your pectorals, especially at the end of the range of motion where you are usually weakest. Flyes define and shape. Don't use a lot of weight because you'll risk injury. I do four sets of 15–20 repetitions on the pec-deck. Study my exercise section *closely.*

The dumbbell pull-over is a great exercise that almost all "experts" ignore. Too bad. It's a wonderful finishing exercise for your pectorals, lats, deltoids and abdominal muscles! Concentrate on form with a slight elbow bend. I do three sets of 15 repetitions.

Another finishing exercise for your pectorals is the cable crossover (you can do it one- or two-handed). I do them slowly. Crossovers don't mean using bench-press weights. Use medium weights and good form. Using a slow, continuous tension movement gives you definition and shape. I do two sets of 25 reps!

In my current chest workout, I do 20–26 sets. That's a lot of sets. Remember, I have been at this now for 12 years. I was always known as a bodybuilder who did a lot of sets, yet most of my workouts aren't high set. Training chest (compared to legs) is always fun.

SHOULDERS

People ask me where I get energy to train. I follow my inclinations, which means

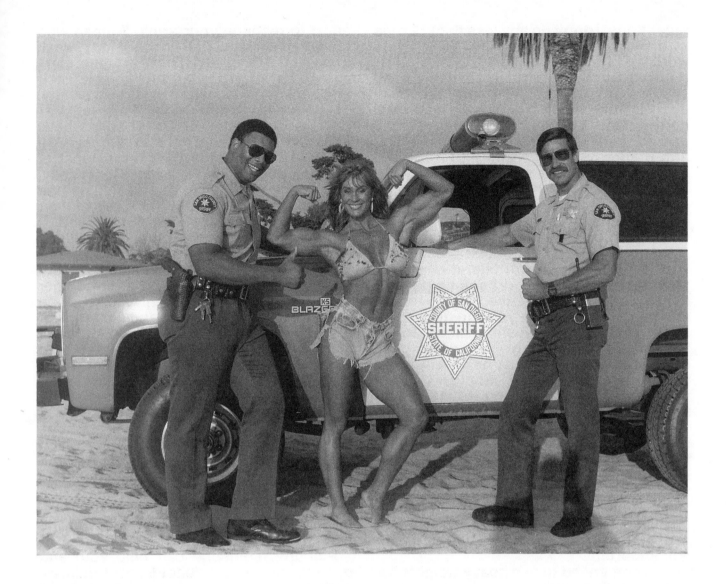

Cory looks "arresting" in this photo—at least San Diego's finest seem to think so.

working out is a matter of heart and mind. Sweat and strain don't bother me. My energy is always there. As I go into the gym with any particular body part in mind to train, my heart takes over. Working out means doing, not sitting and thinking about it.

One thing: If you find that your workout saps your drive and energy, dump it for a different workout. The ultimate workout is still the one that works for you. Do what your body responds to, regardless of what is supposed to be right according to some expert. That is the most expert advice I can give you! This is my approach to shoulder training and all other body areas.

My Favorite Shoulder Exercises

Presses are the best exercises for strengthening, shaping and toning your shoulder muscles. It doesn't matter much which particular pressing exercise you do either. Dumbbells, barbells or machine presses all work your deltoids well.

However, the behind-the-neck press can be a troublemaker, so it might cause discomfort or pain for some of you. If so, use dumbbells or barbells in front presses.

Presses are good because they work your deltoids, upper pectorals, triceps and upper-back muscles. Because of this multiple muscle involvement, I almost always train my shoulders along with my chest.

I like to use dumbbells. Dumbbells are more natural and unrestricted than barbells. I start with light weights for 20 reps and then go heavier on my sets for 12–15 repetitions. I don't do any less than 12 reps with dumbbell presses. Four to six sets work well for me.

I like seated lateral raises. When you sit you're less likely to swing the dumbbells up by leaning forward and using backward body motion. You must isolate your medial deltoid muscles, which produce lateral arm motion. So sit upright and raise and lower the dumbbells slowly. I have always liked 4 or 5 sets of 10–15 repetitions best, right after my dumbbell presses. I like lateral raises so much though that I've also done them before presses.

You can't just do dumbbell presses for your anterior deltoids or lateral raises for your medial deltoids without doing rear raises (these are also called bent-over lateral or rear raises) for your posterior deltoids. With shoulder development, go for beauty and proportion! You don't have eyes in the back of your head, but don't forget the backs of your shoulders! I do 4 or 5 sets of rear raises for 10–15 repetitions.

When I was competing in 1988, I did shrugs for the first time to fill in my upper trapezius from the front. Your trapezius are important muscles. That's not to say I think women bodybuilders should have necks like former football player Lyle Alzado. I never desired a thick neck (nor do most women). However, toned neck muscles are still important.

You don't need to use heavy weights for shrugs. Using heavy weights keeps you from working your shoulders through a full range of motion. I do shrugs with wrist straps to help my grip and I do 3 or 4 sets of 10–15 repetitions. I don't use a pyramid method. I just use a fixed weight for my repetitions.

The wide-shoulder/narrow-hip look is still in. Cable raises not only give you constant tension through a maximum range of motion, but the tension increases as you move farther through the range of motion. Cables are great because you can start in front or behind your body to stress your deltoid muscles differently. I do 4 or 5 sets of 12–20 repetitions.

Altogether, I do 19–25 sets for shoulders, usually after my chest workout, although sometimes I reverse the order. Most women can't do enough shoulder work!

Believe it or not, it doesn't require much effort to reshape your arms. Women who are out of shape usually have skinny, weak arms and tire easily. These women can't carry a bag of groceries a half block. Their arms are gross because they're so skinny. They look like Olive Oyl in "Popeye."

Or, women who are out of shape have arms that look like Brutus in "Popeye." If they're overweight in their arms, most of it is usually in their triceps. Genetically, men store more fat in their waistline and women store more fat in the backs of their arms and this can get way out of hand.

It's easier to tone up and firm skinny arms than it is to reduce chubby arms, but both goals can be accomplished with some effort in the gym and at the dinner table. If you are overweight you must do extra things (like aerobics and dieting), not just direct arm exercise. Since you can't spot reduce exclusively in any one area (remove fat completely from one body area without also losing some fat from other areas of your body), you have to establish a real fat-burning lifestyle.

In either case (skinny-minnie or chubby), to tone up, get firmness, shape and strength into your arms, pull-ups and push-ups are a start. They're better than doing curls with the family dictionary or a Bible! However, pull-ups are not easy, especially if you're overweight. Most of the time, they're impossible.

Pull-ups (someone can help you) and push-ups tone your deltoids, pectorals, biceps and triceps. But, if you did just three sets of dumbbell curls and dumbbell tricep extensions with progressively heavier weights (for 15–20 reps each), you'd quickly reshape your arms because your arms respond to weight training exercise better than any other body part.

My Favorite Arm Exercises

Alternate dumbbell curls are kind of fun (as fun as any exercise can be). This is my favorite bicep exercise that can be used for size- or strength-building or shaping and refining. I work up to a fairly heavy weight for 10–15 repetitions. I've used 50-pound dumbbells, but this exercise must

All you need to get in this kind of shape is the will and the workout!

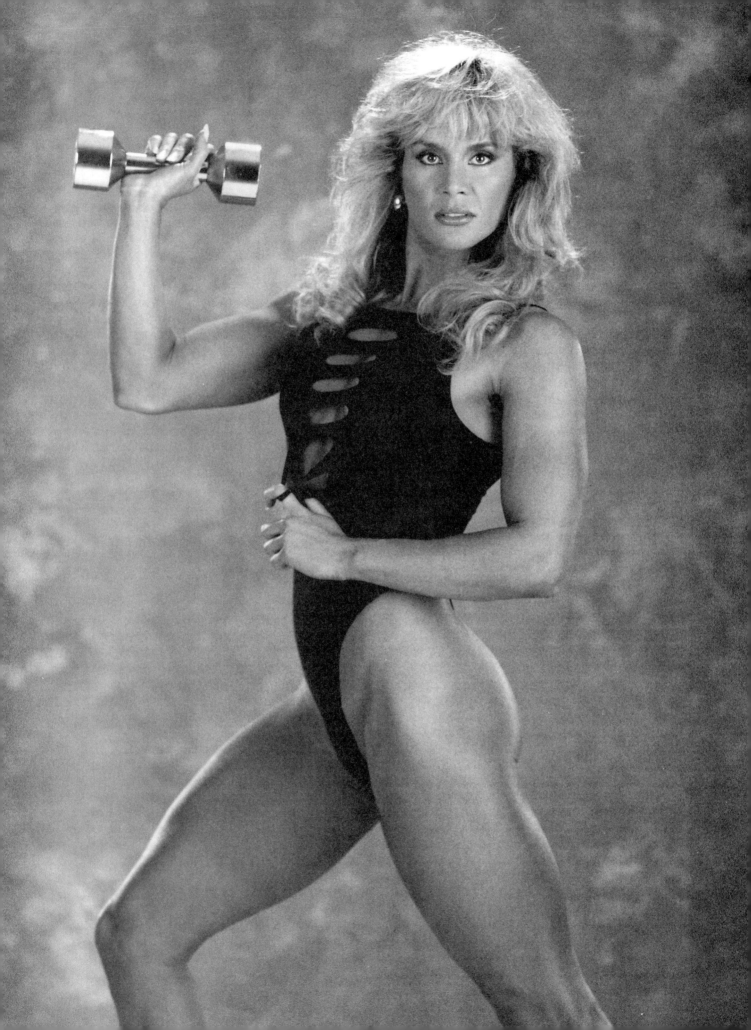

be done with good technique to be effective. Otherwise, your upper back and shoulder muscles do too much of the work. Generally, I do 4–6 sets of 10–15 repetitions using a pyramid method.

I do five sets of barbell curls starting with 25 reps and going backward: 20, 15, and two sets of 10 reps. On each set I use heavier weights. I usually use a straight bar but once in a while, the EZ-curl bar. Standing barbell curls are one of the best exercises for bigger biceps (thin women pay attention)! Why so much emphasis on pyramids? Pyramids provide a gradual warm-up, which helps avoid injuries. Variability in reps with heavy and lighter weights works all aspects of your muscle cells.

The Scott curl adds an interesting angle to arm shaping. Use either a barbell, dumbbell or cable. The cable is probably the most effective because it provides continuous tension through the whole motion (this is unlike barbells and dumbbells, which get easier toward the very end of the range of motion). The forward tilt of your upper arms stresses your large brachialis muscles overlying your elbow joints. Don't go too fast on this exercise and don't try to use too much weight. Lower your weights very slowly and carefully because there's a stretch on your biceps tendon in the down position. I like to do four sets of 15 repetitions in the Scott curl using a fixed weight without pyramids.

Concentration curls give good muscle isolation. You don't have too much strength in the concentration curl position. Concentrate to make your reps and don't use too much weight (either with dumbbells or on the cables). This is my final biceps exercise and I do 3 or 4 sets of 10–12 repetitions. I don't recommend pyramiding with concentration curls.

I do only three exercises for my triceps because my years of pressing exercises have firmed them pretty well. Unfortunately, your triceps are muscles where results don't seem to keep up with your efforts (like calves). So, I only do what I need to keep them sharp.

The triceps push-down on the lat machine using pyramids is my favorite. These have given me strength, size, firmness, and defined shape. I like to do 4 or 5 sets of 10–15 repetitions. On the end rep of each of my sets, I do a hard flex (in the extended position). This seems to firm and sharpen my triceps. Remember, if your triceps are fatty you have to use high reps and very little rest between sets, if any at all. Train with a circuit arm routine and keep your fat intake down.

You can do triceps extensions lying, sitting or standing. Triceps extensions stress the long head of your three-headed triceps muscle, which means they will add thickness and strength. I do the same here, 4 or 5 sets of 10–15 repetitions with a fixed weight. Read more about this great exercise in my how-to chapter!

Another favorite of mine is the dumbbell or cable kickback. I usually do this exercise with my elbow fixed (just moving my forearm backward), but lately I've experimented with straight-arm kickbacks which affects my muscles differently. This is a tough isolation exercise and I do 3 or 4 sets of 10–15 repetitions with a fixed weight.

I'm not a fan of big, thick forearms on women, but I want functional strength in my forearms. You should have enough forearm and hand strength to use a tire wrench to turn the lug nuts on a hubcap if you need to change a tire, and be able to unscrew jar caps. When I work my forearms, it's always after biceps and triceps. If you work your forearms before your biceps and triceps, your grip will be shot and you might not be able to work your biceps and triceps at all! I do 2 or 3 sets of 15–20 in the reverse curl. You also need strong forearms and wrists for many sports.

Because reverse curls work my forearm extensors so well, I usually do only regular (forward) wrist curls with my hands supinated (palms up). This exercise works your forearm flexor muscles. A couple of sets of 20 reps are fine. However, if you like to play golf, tennis or softball, do a few more sets.

I vary my exercises, sets and reps when I train my arms. Sometimes I work my triceps and biceps together with some forearm work at the end. At other times, I train my biceps with back and triceps with chest and shoulders. Again, it doesn't do much good to know these individual body-part exercises without knowing how to put

Cory doesn't "kneel down" to body fat with age. Even women in their forties and beyond can benefit from Cory Everson's Workout.

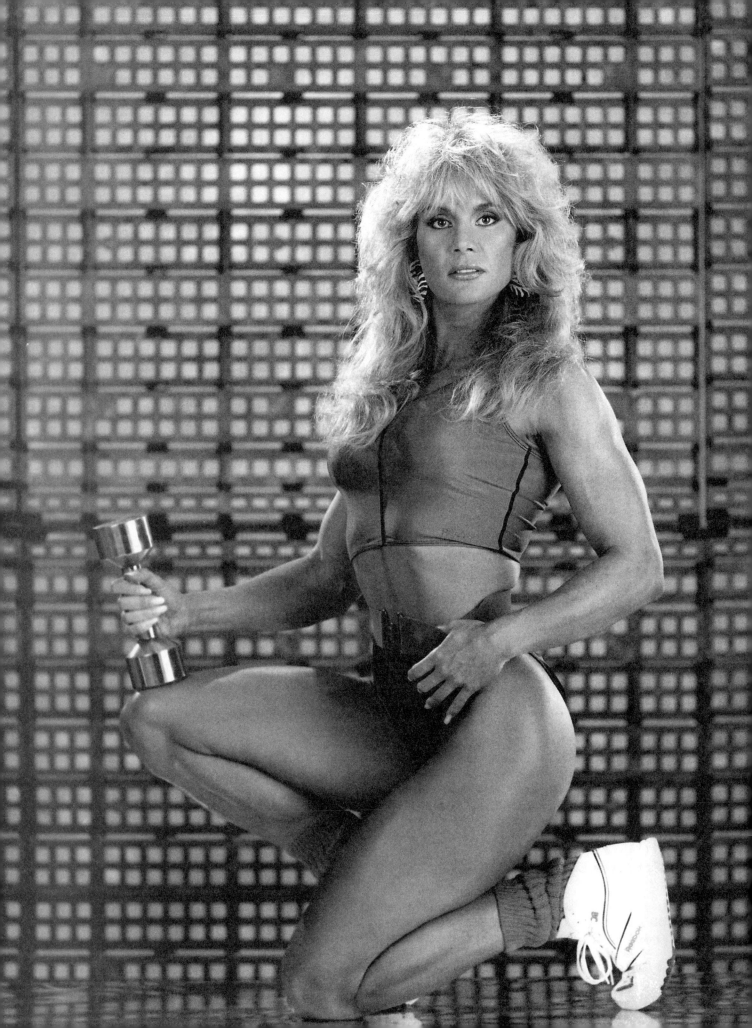

them together in an effective routine, and that's coming up!

BACK

Last year, a *Time* magazine poll showed that only four out of five American teenagers know enough geography to correctly identify the United States on a map! Thirty-four percent couldn't pick out the Pacific Ocean. Balboa would turn over in his grave.

Speaking of geography, did you know that there are at least 15 different muscles that attach to your back scapulae (shoulder blades)? These include your rhomboids; upper, middle and lower trapezius; levator scapulae; serratus interior; pectoralis minor; deltoids; supraspinatus; infraspinatus; subscapularis; teres minor and major; biceps short and long heads; coracobrachialis and triceps long head.

Add to that list of back muscles your latissimus, erector spinae and your deep back muscles and that is a wonderful, complicated piece of geography! You don't have to be a professor of earth science at Yale to get a good back workout, but by having an understanding of your back geography, you'll understand better why it is necessary to do a variety of back exercises for complete development.

What Beginners Should Do

Beginners (six months or less training) should do four basic back exercises. This is more than for other body parts. The four are: lat machine pull-downs to the front, bent-over rows with either dumbbells or a barbell, assisted pull-ups and hyperextensions to just beyond parallel position. Intermediate trainees (six months to a year) should add long pulley rows and shrugs. And advanced trainees can add flat-back deadlifts.

My Favorite Back Exercises

Even though pull-ups (hands pronated, palms away) are difficult, especially if you are overweight, they develop your latissimus muscles. A good spotter can help you up, allowing you to concentrate on your back muscles and not your arm muscles. Your spotter should aid you just enough to make the repetition. Your spotter should not "lift" you up. You have to do the work. Because pull-ups are so hard, do as many as you can by yourself and then do more reps with the help of your spotter. Make sure you get up to four sets of 10–15 repetitions (if your spotter can make it)!

The lat machine pull-down is an exercise of art and science. And, it is one of the most abused exercises in the gym. Because your lats extend your shoulder joints, you have to get your elbows behind your body at all finishing points in all your back exercises. If you don't do this, you won't work your lats effectively. Study my exercise descriptions and pictures in my special chapter on this. Don't round over on your pull-downs because you will substitute other muscles for your lats. I like to do 4–6 sets of 10–15 repetitions using a pyramid method.

Of the barbell bent row and dumbbell row, I like the dumbbell row better because your lower back is protected from injury. When you support your body with your knee on a bench (refer to descriptions), stress is removed from your lower back. Use a reasonable weight for these, but range of motion and technique are more important. I do 3–5 sets of 10–12 repetitions, usually with a fixed weight.

The long pulley row works your upper-back muscles closer to your spine. It will also work your biceps. This is one reason to work your back and arm flexor muscles in the same workout. Use fairly heavy weights, but do not swing the weights up or round your back over during the extended position. I like to do about 4 or 5 sets of 10–15 repetitions, using a pyramid method.

Don't be afraid of the "hyper" in front of the word "extension." Although doctors tell us never to hyperextend our spines, the word in weight training is kind of a misnomer as in this exercise (hyperextension), you start in full flexion and extend to a parallel position (or just a bit beyond, so there's only a little "hyper" in the extension).

This works your erector spinae muscles directly without strain on your spinal ligaments and connective tissues. I like to do

2 or 3 sets of 20 repetitions without adding any extra resistance.

Your Lower Back

Very few people are fortunate enough to go through life without injuring their lower back. If you have a weak lower back or pain in your lower back, please refer to the suggested lower-back workout in the special conditions section of my book.

God created us with our eyes in front of our body so we can see only forward. That being the case, don't ignore what's behind you, especially your back development.

After seeing this photo, the phrase "on the rocks" shouldn't have anything to do with beverages!

THE MIDDLE CLASS WITH NO CLASS IN THEIR MIDDLE! TRAINING YOUR ABDS!

Most of my book sections focus on women's problems. This time, however, my comments will be directed to both sexes and even more so to you guys! When it comes to exercising and eating properly to avoid becoming a veritable jelly belly with age, men (and women) need to pay attention to my abdominal workouts.

There are many different opinions about controlling middle-age spread, but simple exercises and low-fat eating are the keys. Remember from my earlier discussions that not only does performing muscle work actually burn calories and fat, but the very nature of having muscle also burns calories due to an increased metabolic rate.

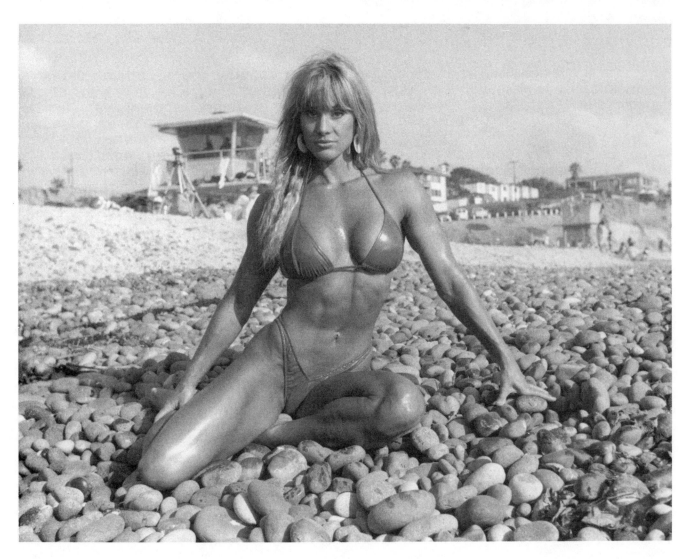

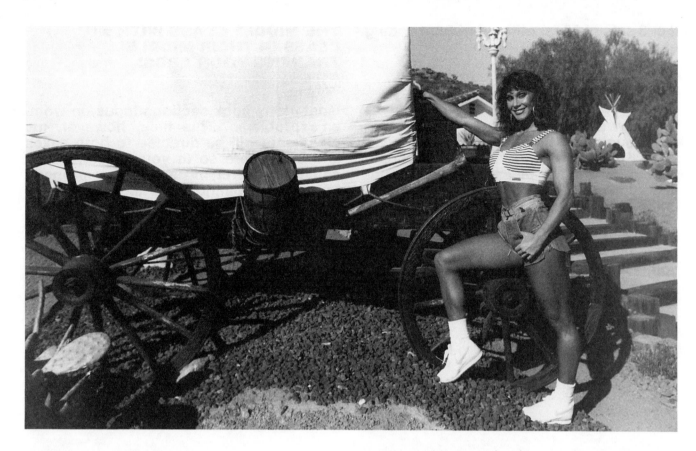

Always the unique designer, Cory commissioned a Western artisan to make a covered wagon for her front yard!

When people say you can't burn fat through abdominal exercises, they are both correct and incorrect.

Dropping Fat

You need to expend calories to burn fat, and you need to build up your muscles to burn fat, and abdominal exercises can help with that. As you should know by now, you need both aerobic and anaerobic exercises to really get a handle on those love handles—and don't let anyone tell you different. Doing exercises to shed fat everywhere (biking, swimming, fast walking, jogging, etc.) is crucial, but so are specific abdominal exercises.

I have strong opinions on abdominal development. I like to work my abdominals five times a week and I think you should too, whether you are a beginner or advanced trainee. Work them consistently at the same time each day. Start by working your obliques first.

Your obliques (outer abdominals) have much better endurance than your rectus abdominis (inner abdominals). Isolate your abdominals as much as possible. Your hip flexors work in unison with your abdominals. In fact, your hip flexors are often strong and overdeveloped relative to your abdominals. If this is the case and you start an abdominal routine that is slipshod, not only will you fail to improve the strength, shape and firmness of your abdominals, but you may fatigue your hip muscles or worse yet, end up with a slipshod lower back from injury!

My Favorite Abdominal Exercises

If you follow a straight set system, work your obliques first. This is not as important if you train in a circuit system, which most people like to do (nonstop abdominal circuits). With someone anchoring your legs, the side sit-up is effective at working your obliques. I do four sets of 25–50 repetitions for each side without rest. I like side sit-ups better than the more conventional side bends with dumbbells.

Leg raises do work your hip flexors, but by doing them right, you'll isolate your rectus and transversus abdominis muscles as much as possible. Study carefully my exercise description and do at least four sets of 20–50 repetitions.

The crunch is the best overall abdominal exercise and if you had time to do only one exercise *in your life,* make this the one! It is so good because it works your abdominals best. Strong, conditioned abdominals prevent back problems, help posture and prevent you from getting Dunlop's disease (that's the condition where your belly dun-lops over your belt)! There's a trick or two to doing crunches right so pay special attention to this exercise description too. I recommend four sets of 15–50 slow, controlled repetitions five days a week.

Some people have very strong abdominal muscles or they want to make them strong and/or thicker. It's hard to overload your abdominals in the crunch exercise. There's no effective way to hold heavy weights behind your head and do half sit-ups! What to do? Pull-down crunches. On this machine, you can do a reverse crunch with as much weight as you want. Pull off to the sides to work your obliques too. I do 2 or 3 sets of 10–15 repetitions, with weight, using a pyramid method.

The incline sit-up is an advanced exercise. Try it once you've developed good strength in your abdominals and flexibility in your hip flexors. You also need a strong, healthy lower back! For maximum development though, this is the exercise that will do it! I like to do one set of 100 reps. On my first 50 reps I hold a 10-pound weight plate. I then drop it off and do another 50 reps. Work up to it.

Every "expert" advises against doing twisting, sighting dangers to your spine. However, they all do the exercise wrong. Twisting sit-ups can be dangerous if you do them too fast or twist too far to the side each time. Plus, if you twist while sitting upright you do absolutely nothing to condition your abdominals since you are not twisting against any resistance!

To be effective, you have to have your legs anchored and lean backward and then twist *very slowly* while "flexing" your obliques hard at the end of each twist. Experiment with this exercise to see if you like it. I do 2 or 3 sets of 25 reps on each side.

Here's one for you—the Cory Pushaway. This is a tricep and abdominal exercise.

Learn how to *push yourself away* from the dinner table when desserts and extra helpings are offered!

Are You a Pear or an Apple?

You women who are so concerned with extra fat in your hips and rear should feel good about at least one scientific fact. Women who are built like pears (with extra weight in their hips and rear end) are *less* likely to suffer heart attacks, strokes or diabetes than women who are built like apples, with more weight stored in their abdominals. I suppose the major reason for this is that having some extra weight in your lower extremities is a virtue of heredity, related to childbirth, while extra stomach fat is not.

Closer analysis shows that extra abdominal fat in men and women is not subcutaneous (directly under your skin). Instead, this fat is behind the muscle cavity wall, inside the abdominal cavity around internal, visceral organs. That's dangerous fat, while subcutaneous fat (usually the kind women store in their hips), is not. That is not to say that it makes women happy to have it there! But at least you won't die from it!

WHR

You should pay close attention to your waist-to-hip ratio (WHR). This ratio should be less than one, or better yet, less than .85. If your waist is 30″, then your hips should be at least 34–35 inches. It should not be the other way around. Your waist should not be bigger, or as big as your hips. Here's a way to figure your ratio: Waist measurement divided by hip measurement times 100. If this is less than 85 you are okay!

You'll see in my workout section that I recommend training your abdominals in nonstop circuits of 3–6 exercises for 15–50 repetitions, in most cases. Besides direct abdominal exercises, the other factors in slimming a jelly belly are twofold. Do some aerobics every day (30–60 minutes) and greatly reduce the fatty foods you eat—every day!

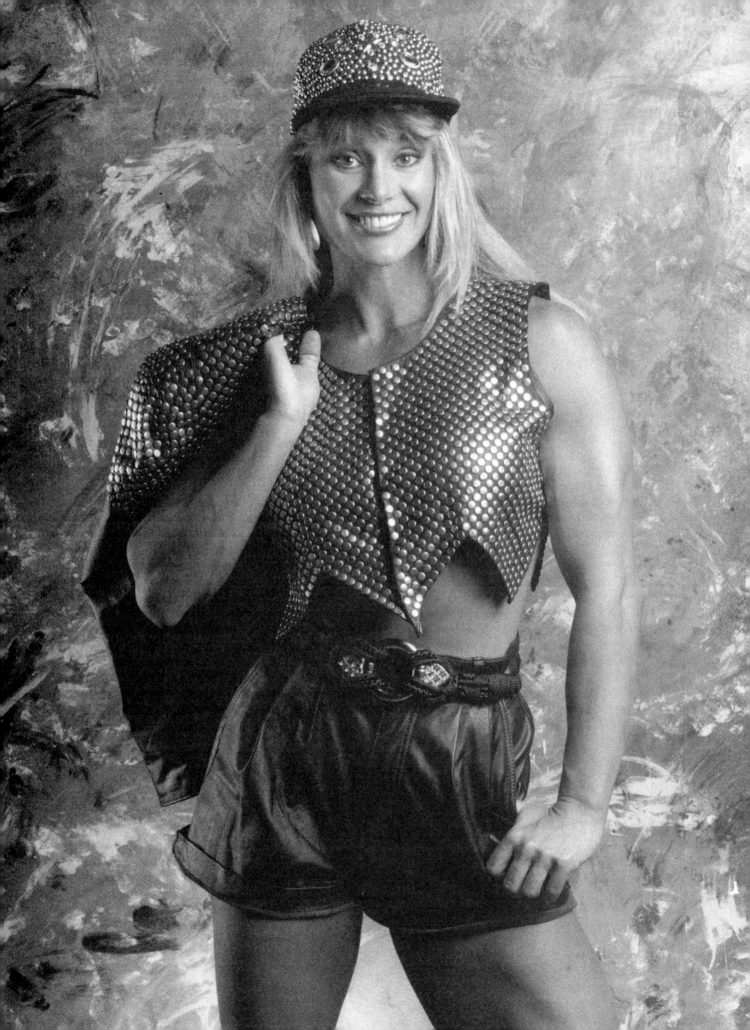

6
WORKING YOUR LOWER BODY

THE REAL BATTLE OF THE BULGE!

I meet too many women locked in a frustrating battle to slim, shape and firm their hips, thighs and glutes. Those of you lucky enough not to have this problem can't imagine how frustrated so many of these women are. It's frustrating to me too because I know that heredity sometimes seems to override everything, including physiological logic! But, I also know that many women exercise incorrectly or incompletely and that's where I can help.

One thing you can see about competitive bodybuilders—they have the firmest glutes, thighs and hips in the business. Bodybuilders, sprinters, jumpers and runners always have tight, shapely glutes, hips and upper thighs. There are reasons—not just heredity! It's the type of exercises bodybuilders do (and how they do them) and the diets they follow.

I know several top professional bodybuilders who didn't have small, tight hips and glutes before they got into bodybuilding. Weight training and good nutrition

gave them a complete makeover—better than any plastic surgeon could do in 10 years of surgery. I know it can be done and you and I will do it together!

At the same time, I'm not dumb enough to think we are all the same. Some of you were born with more fat cells in your hips and upper thighs. Some of you have metabolic rates slower than molasses in a Vermont January! Some of you were born of energetic parents, raised in a high-energy/activity athletic-peer-group environment. If so, you're lucky. You have a short time advantage in staying firm lasting into early adulthood (even if you do nothing after high school), but it won't last forever.

Even though my workouts are devoted to shaping up, maintain a good image of yourself, even if you're not in the shape right now that you want to be in. Although at times it might not seem so, there are worse things in life than fat hips! Nevertheless, I'll attack the problem as if it's the most pressing issue of your life.

SOMATOTYPES

A clothing and interior designer, Cory appreciates stylish clothing. So do we.

Besides sex and genetic body fat problems, there's another factor in your battle

125

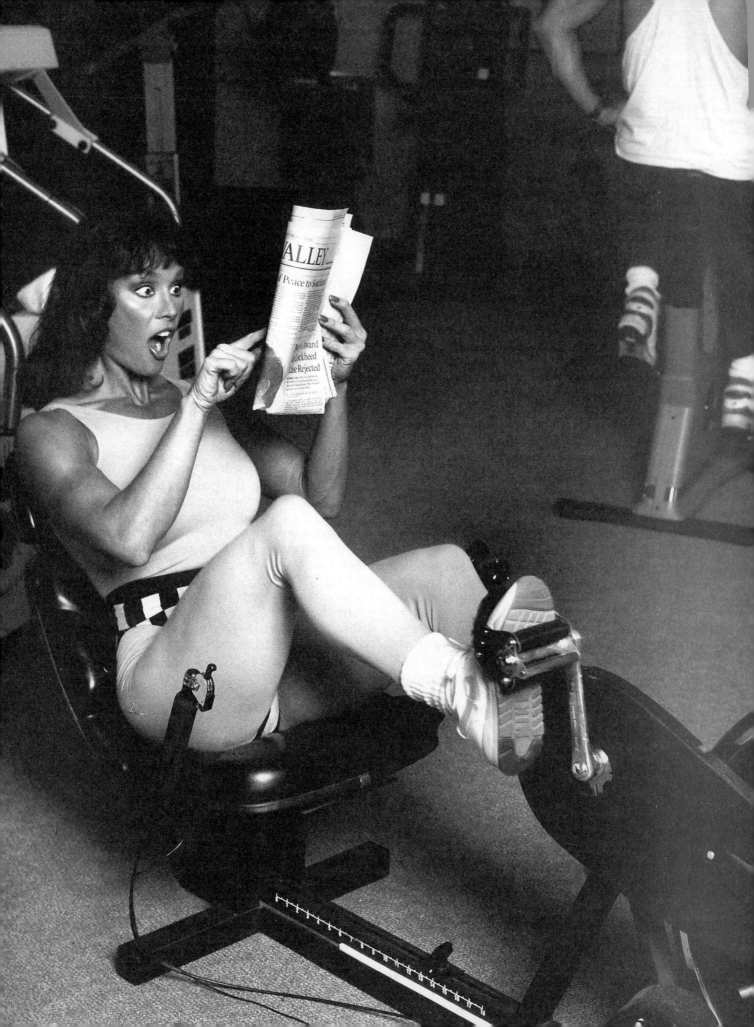

to shape up your lower body. Somatotype refers to your natural body build. Your somatotype partially determines your response to exercise and diet.

If you have a slight frame and can eat ice cream until the cows come home without putting on a pound, you are probably an ectomorph with a fast metabolism. Ectomorphs have a terribly tough time gaining weight and muscle and they usually don't have problems with heart disease. If this is you, your diet has to be calorically dense and you can't weight train or do aerobics as often, or do as many exercises as most people. In fact, aerobics are pretty much out altogether. You need to save the calories!

On the other hand, if you take a sniff of chocolate cake and the next day your pants don't fit, you're likely an endomorph. An endomorph usually is overweight, has big bones and a slow metabolism. Endomorphs gain weight on tuna fish if they don't exercise. You might have a life battling the bulge if you don't concentrate on putting the exercise/diet hammer to the metal all the time. It doesn't exactly make for a fun time at the dinner table, unless you exercise regularly, hard and right.

If you have average-size bones and are naturally strong and muscular, call yourself a mesomorph. You are genetically blessed. Mesomorphs can usually eat a lot without gaining fat. When mesomorphs exercise for three months, they gain as much muscle as the average person does after exercising for a year.

So, we have different genetic structures, metabolic rates and activity levels. Nothing about that precludes you from improving yourself. It might be harder for you than for some, but you can succeed nonetheless.

What woman doesn't want to improve the shape of her legs, glutes and hips? Even trim women want to. Despite your condition, don't give up the good fight. If you're not happy with your current condition and if you haven't exercised and you live on potato chips, then get off your fatty acid and do something about it before you have a massive coronary.

I'm supposed to be using the recumbent cycle, but someone wrote in the paper that I might lose the Ms. Olympia contest. Imagine.

CIRCUIT SETS

In terms of shaping and firming your legs, hips and glutes, I recommend weight-training circuits. Circuit sets are a part of my triangle of fitness—area-specific aerobics, circuit weight workouts and low-fat dieting. Specific fat-burning aerobics conditions your heart, burns off body fat *and* directly works your hip, upper-thigh and glute muscles while it pumps up your heart and burns body fat.

The best aerobics? I think hill walking is tops because of the intensity (and the outdoor environment). Following trudging up hills: repetitive interval sprinting (alternating sprinting 50 yards and fast-walking 100 yards for 20–40 minutes), cross-country skiing, fast-walking up slight hills, stair climbing, outdoor biking over uneven terrain and indoor stationary biking where you can also pump your arms as you ride and a vigorous step-aerobic program.

These aerobics work your glutes, hips and upper thighs well. They're more effective for this than swimming, jogging, rope skipping and aerobic dance, for instance.

You have to learn how to eat right. Refer to my nutrition chapters to learn about low-fat eating and proper nutrition. Without it, any exercise program will only do half the job!

Weight exercises should be nonstop or with very little rest between them. Of course, if you are a beginner and not in good shape, it's impossible to do your workout without rest unless you only do *one* set. And that won't get you anywhere. Don't try to set any world records at first. You must start slowly and work your way up.

I recently read about a man so obese (he weighed 925 pounds) that he had to lose 200 pounds just so he could finally get out of bed! He probably burned 1,000 calories the day he sat up and got out of bed. He went very slowly with diet and exercise because he was so far gone (almost all the way).

With weight training, the best way to work stubborn hips, thighs and glutes is to do 4–6 exercises in a row. I call this a circuit giant set (not because you have giant thighs, but because there are so many exercises in one set).

Believe me, training with giant sets in

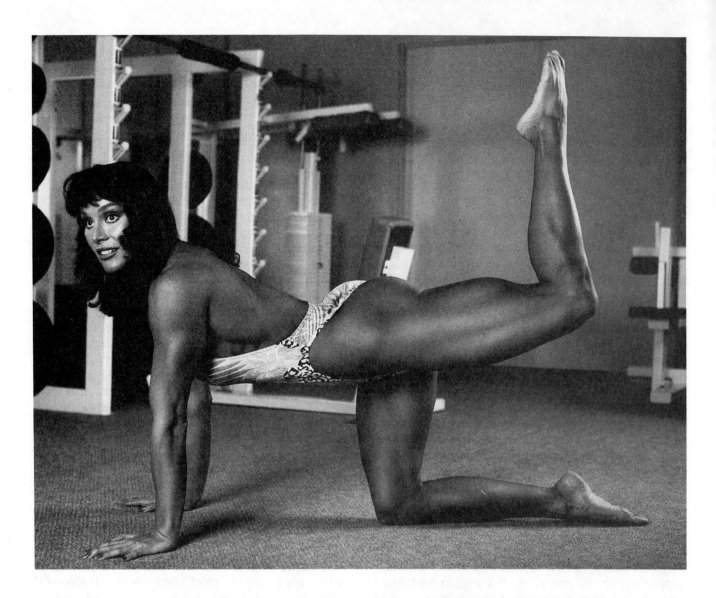

Hip extensions with a bent knee shift some of the stress from your hamstrings to your gluteus muscles.

HIP HELPERS/BUN BURNERS/THIGH TIGHTENERS: THE FIRST STEP

circuit format is hard. It burns calories big time and shapes you up fast! However, it's easy for overweight people to overtrain, in spite of all their stored fat for energy, so don't overdo it. Competitive bodybuilders do giant sets before competition to "train down" and, literally, overtrain. It's not a training system that an ectomorph does to gain weight.

So, my three-tiered approach to fat-burning and muscle toning flabby areas is giant-set weight circuits, specific glute/hip/thigh aerobics (4–6 days a week) and low-fat, calorically balanced, nutritionally correct eating *at all times.*

Beginners should spend time on the floor exercising in natural motions. Do leg abduction, adduction, flexion and extension exercises without weights. Most beginners just use the weight of their legs as resistance. Some of you might be able to start with ankle weights right away.

In "Putting It All Together" there's a separate leg workout for real beginners—starting with the weight of your legs, some other free-lance exercises like lunges and squats (body weight as resistance) and then followed with most of the same exercises using ankle weights.

However, soon enough you will be ready for a more advanced hip/glute/thigh-shaping program, a harder, more effective workout. I have a specific program for you, in four steps. The first step is free-form exercise. The second step utilizes pulleys. Even if you're really out of shape, you still should be ready for the second step after spending about three months on the beginning workout.

Beginning exercises are free leg flexion, extension (with and without flexed knees), abduction, adduction, lunge, body extension, squat and calf raise. You do these exercises at least five days a week, in addition to your specific aerobics. You do 3–5 giant sets and all the exercises should be done for 25 repetitions.

INTERMEDIATE HIP/GLUTE/THIGH SHAPING: THE SECOND STEP

In this workout, you train your hips, thighs and glutes four times a week: Monday, Wednesday, Friday and Saturday, for instance. On Tuesday, Thursday, Saturday and Sunday, you walk hills or do your favorite aerobic exercise. Every day, eat correctly. The big difference between this and the beginner program is that you add resistance to all your exercises and you lower your repetitions, which builds your muscles more.

Instead of sets of 25 repetitions, do 15–20 repetitions (work to failure, or until you can't do another repetition of that exercise) on each exercise, one set of each, one right after the other, to make a complete giant set. Repeat your giant sets 3–5 times! It won't be easy.

Get used to flexing, extending and squeezing your muscles at the end of each repetition. You need strong, concentrated muscle contractions to firm your muscles faster and to control your muscles.

A nonstop circuit giant-set workout for at least 45 minutes burns 300–500 calories a day; aerobics burns another 300–500 calories each day; and cut at least 250 daily fat calories from your diet. This guarantees a weight loss of 1 to 2 pounds each week. Losing a pound per week is the safest and most effective way to get a long-term weight loss.

INTERMEDIATE HIP/GLUTE/THIGH SHAPING: THE THIRD STEP

It'll happen sooner than you think. One day those pulley exercises will be easy. It's time to change. The two changes in your program are exercises and number of weight workout days. Use weights three days a week. Don't get the idea though that your weight training portion of the triangle is easier because you dropped back from four workout days to three. On the contrary, it's going to be much *harder* because the exercises take *more* effort and energy. Continue to do 3–5 giant sets, but now 10–15 reps.

Third-Step Giant-Set Exercises

Refer to my exercise chapter to learn how to do all your exercises. At this point in the workout, start with the squat. Squatting is the best overall exercise for your hips, glutes and thighs. It's good for your lower-back muscles (provided you have a healthy lower back to begin with). Yes, it does build hip, thigh and glute muscle, but so what? It's muscle so it's firm flesh. And squats make your glutes tighter, rounder and firmer, not wider.

Squats are *not* bad for your knees, provided you don't drop into a deep position and bounce out of the bottom. If you raise your heels with a 2–3″ board and keep your seat tucked in (instead of pushing it out like a power lifter does), with minimal upper-body forward lean, your glutes will stay round and firm, your hips and upper thighs strong and slender.

Flat-footed squatting also works your glutes, but gives you heavier development in your lower glute fibers. Wider-stance squatting works too. Vary your style (including using the Smith Machine) to work your hips, upper thighs and glutes from all angles.

When bodybuilding, I treated the squat as a separate entity, but for slimming and shaping problem areas, don't use the conventional set system of squatting. That's for power, strength and muscle size. Instead, make them your first and hardest exercise in a giant-set circuit. Do 15–18 repetitions for all your sets.

People forget the leg press to slim their hips and tighten their glutes, but it's direct and very effective, especially if you place your feet "up and out" on the foot board as you press. Do your reps slowly and strictly as explained in my exercise section. Vary your foot position and do higher reps, in the 20–25 range.

The step-up was popular years ago, faded for a while and now is making a significant impact again on shaping and slimming glutes, upper thighs and hips. Use steps or benches of varying height, from 4–20". I like to step up all my reps on one leg before moving to my other leg. Do 3–5 giant sets of 15–20 reps each leg. Don't use any weight to start, but gradually work up to light dumbbells or a free bar with weight.

Lunges are a great exercise. Study my exercise description in the next chapter. I lunge slowly. You can go up on your toes each rep. On the way back down, you can stop at parallel or go deeper. Do 15–20 lunges for each leg. Lunges are probably safer and easier than step-ups, but don't use bars or dumbbells until you've mastered technique.

For a special effect, do lunges onto a step or stair. Do them very slowly and go all the way up on your toes for your calves.

The leg curl is the most overlooked and underrated exercise for firming your upper thighs and backside. Both standing and lying leg curls do the job well. You work your hamstrings as a hip extensor and knee flexor and your glutes in their role of hip extensor, especially if at the end of your curl you "try" to lift your whole hip up and back, giving a supercontraction of your glutes. Do 15–20 reps in each as part of your 3–5 giant sets.

The leg extension is the old standby for muscle development around your knees. No one looks good with either bony *or* fat knees. Leg extensions firm your thighs. Don't use a lot of weight, just do them strictly. Go for a high repetition pump with about 20 reps and flex your muscles very hard at the end. Leg extensions will balance out your hamstring development.

There are a few exercises I missed: hack squats, hyperextensions and donkey calf raises—they're coming up!

ADVANCED HIP/GLUTE/THIGH SHAPING: THE FOURTH STEP

For advanced thigh shape and definition you have to use a novel approach. Unfortunately, it's not enough to do regular squats, leg extensions and leg curls, even if you're doing intense giant sets. These exercises, along with aerobics and low-fat foods, help a tremendous amount, making you more defined and less fat, but for a woman with real problem areas, you need more.

Developing thigh definition requires muscle control. You don't get thigh definition unless you can control your muscles. What I mean by this is if you have extreme thigh definition when your legs are relaxed, you're too skinny, girl! To develop thigh-muscle control, do a variety of exercises and learn how to bring your muscle definition out through muscle control.

Specific exercises I use to get thigh definition are slow squats using the Smith Machine (with or without your heels raised); leg presses with your feet close together and down low on the foot board; hack squats, also with your feet close together and low on the foot board; slow leg extensions with a two-second squeeze of your thigh muscles at the full extension position; slow step-ups; Cory lunges (stepping backward instead of forward); hyperextensions and donkey calf raises.

Putting these exercises into the giant-set format means more hard work. Refer to the exercise descriptions and workout chapter for all the juicy details!

Keep your aerobics going. Do them six days a week with variety. Try hill walking three times, biking twice and fast-walking once. Mix it up for fun. Besides the weight circuits, aerobics and good nutrition, there's still *more* to do for ultimate thigh, glute and hip definition.

FLEXING AND TENSING FOR ULTIMATE DEFINITION

Bodybuilders have extreme definition during contests for three reasons: low body-fat, a lot of muscle and the ability to *show* these muscles. Bodybuilders spend countless hours learning how to stand, tense and pose to bring out the muscular detail they have worked so hard to develop.

To accomplish this, competitive bodybuilders spend about 20 minutes a day isometrically flexing their muscles. By doing this, you gain control of your thigh muscles and can show specific muscles at will. This trick or technique will help you show (and develop) thigh definition. It's not all for show! Flexing works your muscles very hard and this helps develop definition.

All these great leg exercises will be phased into your overall weight-training workouts coming up! Get ready. I'm not taking any prisoners.

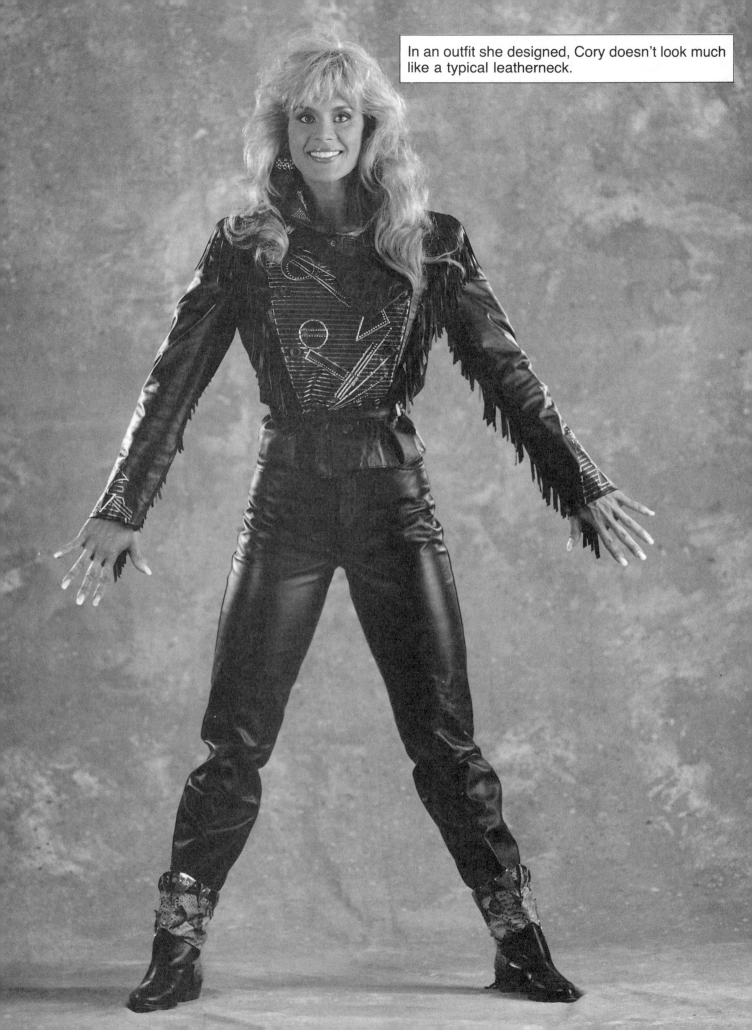

In an outfit she designed, Cory doesn't look much like a typical leatherneck.

7
PUTTING IT ALL TOGETHER

Pearl Buck wrote: "To know what one can have and what to do with it is the basis of equilibrium." I'm telling (and showing) you what you can have. However, knowing what you can have but not knowing what to do with it won't provide equilibrium for your life.

In fact, you can have all the weight-training information in the world, but if you can't put it all together in realistic workouts, you will have no equilibrium and not get any worthwhile results. One of the unfortunate truths about almost all other fitness/bodybuilding books is they don't provide you with enough workout choices. I'm here to see that this won't happen again. Guys and gals, start your engines!

BEGINNING WEIGHT-TRAINING WORKOUTS

Workout Without Weight-Training Equipment (NW)

Mon, Wed and Fri or Tues, Thurs and Sat

Exercise	Sets	Reps
Stretching and Warm-Up		
1. Squat	1–3 ×	10–50
2. Lunge	1–3 ×	10–25
3. Step-Up	1–3 ×	10–25
4. Modified or Regular Push-Up	1–3 ×	5–50
5. Crunch	1–3 ×	10–50
6. Leg Raise	1–3 ×	10–50
7. Floor Hyperextension	1–3 ×	10–20
8. Step or other Aerobics	20–40 minutes	

Beginning Weight-Training Workout (A)

Mon, Wed and Fri or Tues, Thurs and Sat

Exercise	Sets	Reps
Stretching and Warm-Up		
1. Leg Press	1–3 ×	10–20
2. Bench or Incline Dumbbell Press	1–3 ×	10–15
3. Seated Dumbbell Press	1–3 ×	10–15
4. Lat Pull-Down to Front	1–3 ×	10–15
5. Lateral Raise	1–3 ×	10–15
6. Dip	1–3 ×	maximum
7. Barbell Curl	1–3 ×	10–15
8. Leg Extension	1–3 ×	15–20
9. Leg Curl	1–3 ×	15–20
10. Standing Calf Raise	1–3 ×	15–30
11. Crunch	1–3 ×	10–50

Aerobics optional three days a week

Beginning Weight-Training Workout (B)

Mon, Wed and Fri or Tues, Thurs and Sat

Exercise	Sets	Reps
Stretching and Warm-Up		
1. Bench Press	1–3 ×	8–15
2. Leg Press	1–3 ×	12–20
3. Bent-Over Row	1–3 ×	12–20
4. Behind-the-Neck Press	1–3 ×	8–15
5. Lateral Raise	1–3 ×	10–15
6. Bent-Over Dumbbell Raise	1–3 ×	10–20
7. Leg Curl	1–3 ×	10–20
8. Dumbbell Curl	1–3 ×	10–15
9. Tricep Push-Down	1–3 ×	10–15
10. Standing Calf Raise	1–3 ×	15–30
11. Crunch	1–3 ×	10–50

Aerobics optional three days a week

Beginning Weight-Training Workout (C)

Mon, Wed and Fri or Tues, Thurs and Sat

Exercise	Sets	Reps
Stretching and Warm-Up		
1. Incline Press	1–3 ×	8–12
2. Flye	1–3 ×	10–15
3. Machine Press	1–3 ×	8–12
4. Lat Pull-Down to Front	1–3 ×	10–15
5. Lateral Raise	1–3 ×	10–15
6. Seated Pulley Row	1–3 ×	10–15
7. Squat	1–3 ×	10–20
8. Leg Extension	1–3 ×	10–20
9. Leg Curl	1–3 ×	10–20
10. Curl	1–3 ×	10–15
11. Lying Tricep Extension	1–3 ×	10–15
12. Donkey Raise	1–3 ×	12–30
13. Regular Wrist Curl	1–2 ×	20–50
14. Crunch	1–3 ×	10–50

Aerobics optional three days a week

Beginning Weight-Training Workout (D)

Mon, Wed and Fri or Tues, Thurs and Sat

Exercise	Sets	Reps
Stretching and Warm-Up		
1. Squat	2–4 ×	10–20
2. Leg Press	2–4 ×	10–20
3. Bench Press	2–4 ×	10–15
4. Incline Dumbbell Press	2–4 ×	10–15
5. Seated Dumbbell Press	2–4 ×	10–15
6. Shrug	2–4 ×	10–20
7. Scott Curl	1–3 ×	10–15
8. Tricep Push-Down	2–4 ×	10–15
9. Flat-Back Deadlift	1–3 ×	10–15
10. Leg Extension	2–4 ×	10–20
11. Leg Curl	2–4 ×	10–20
12. Donkey Raise	2–4 ×	10–30
13. Reverse Curl	1–3 ×	10–30
14. Crunch	2–4 ×	10–50
15. Lean-Back Twist	1–3 ×	10–50

Aerobics optional three days a week

Beginning Weight-Training Workout (E)

Mon, Wed and Fri or Tues, Thurs and Sat

Exercise	Sets	Reps
Stretching and Warm-Up		
1. Incline Press	2–4 ×	8–12
2. Pec-Deck Flye	1–3 ×	10–20
3. Seated Dumbbell Press	2–4 ×	10–15
4. Front Dumbbell Raise	1–3 ×	10–15
5. Lat Pull-Down to the Front	2–4 ×	10–15
6. Wide-Grip Pull-Up	1–3 ×	maximum
7. Shrug	2–4 ×	10–20
8. EZ-Bar Curl	1–3 ×	10–15
9. Tricep Kickback	1–3 ×	10–15
10. Squat	2–4 ×	10–20
11. Cory Lunge	1–3 ×	10–20
12. Leg Extension	2–4 ×	10–20
13. Standing Leg Curl	1–3 ×	10–20
14. Hyperextension	1–3 ×	10–20
15. Seated Calf Raise	1–3 ×	10–30
16. Crunch	2–4 ×	10–50
17. Side Sit-Up	1–3 ×	10–50

Aerobics optional three days a week

Beginning Weight-Training Workout (F)

Mon and Fri

Exercise	Sets	Reps
Stretching and Warm-Up		
1. Bench Press	1 ×	15
	3 ×	8–10
	1 ×	12–15
2. Behind-the-Neck Press	3 ×	8–10
3. Dip	2–3 ×	maximum
4. Bent-Over Row	2–4 ×	8–12
5. Lat Pull-Down to Front	2–4 ×	8–12
6. Squat	1 ×	15
	3 ×	10–15
7. Leg Extension	3 ×	12
8. Leg Curl	3 ×	12
9. Dumbbell Curl	3 ×	10–12
10. Concentration Curl	2 ×	10–15
11. Tricep Extension	2 ×	10–15
12. Leg Raise	2–4 ×	10–50

Aerobics Optional

Wed

Exercise	Sets	Reps
Stretching and Warm-Up		
1. Incline Press	1 ×	15
	3 ×	10–15
2. Lateral Raise	3 ×	10–15
3. Flat-Back Deadlift	2–3 ×	10–15
4. Leg Press	2–3 ×	10–15
5. Donkey Raise	3 ×	10–30
6. Dumbbell Curl	3 ×	10–15
7. Tricep Pushdown	3 ×	10–15
8. Hyperextension	2–3 ×	10–20
9. Crunch	2–4 ×	10–50

Aerobics Optional

Beginning Weight-Training Workout (G): Weight-Training Workout with Machines (Universal, Eagle, Olympus, etc.)

Mon, Wed and Fri

Exercise	Sets	Reps
Stretching and Warm-Up		
1. Bench Press Station	1–3 ×	10–15
2. Machine Flye Station	1–3 ×	12–20
3. Seated Row Station	1–3 ×	12–20
4. Pull-Over Station	1–3 ×	10–15
5. Shoulder Press Station	1–3 ×	10–15
6. Lateral Raise Station	1–3 ×	12–15
7. Bicep Curl Station	1–3 ×	12–15
8. Tricep Push-Down	1–3 ×	12–15
9. Lat Pull-Down Station	1–3 ×	12–15
10. Leg Press Station	1–3 ×	12–20
11. Leg Extension Station	1–3 ×	10–20
12. Leg Curl Station	1–3 ×	12–20
13. Abdominal Crunch Station	1–3 ×	10–50
14. Back or Hyperextension Station	1–3 ×	10–20

Beginning Weight-Training Workout (H): Emphasis on Weight Reduction/Muscle Toning in your Hips, Glutes and Thighs

Exercise	Sets	Reps
Stretching and Warm-Up		

All exercises performed as a circuit giant set.

	Sets	Reps
1. Squat	1 ×	20
2. Leg Press	1 ×	20
3. Lunge	1 ×	20
4. Step-Up	1 ×	20

Repeat this circuit up to two more times, but *only* after you have adapted to it—after you have done it for at least a month. Start with one set and don't use any weight at all if this is new to you.

	Sets	Reps
5. Cory Lunge	1 ×	20
6. Leg Extension	1 ×	20
7. Leg Curl	1 ×	20
8. Hyperextension	1 ×	15

As above, repeat this circuit up to two more times, but only after a month of doing just one set of each exercise.

	Sets	Reps
9. Smith Rack Squat (non-lockout)	1 ×	20
10. Hack Squat	1 ×	20
11. Standing Calf Raise	1 ×	20
12. Crunch	1 ×	10–50

Cool Down: Because of the aerobic demands of this workout, cool down with walking, light biking and stretching.

Tues, Thurs, Sat and Sun

Stretching and Warm-Up
Aerobics: On each of these days, start slowly and gradually. If you've done nothing before this, start with 10 minutes of walking on flat terrain. Gradually build up until you can do 45 minutes to an hour of fast walking on flat terrain. Work up to hilly terrain. Don't walk all the time. Mix it up. On other days, do The Step workout. Also do stair climbers or stationary bikes (I recommend bikes with arm-working handles) or any aerobics that you enjoy.
Cool Down Stretching

Beginning Weight-Training Workout with Dumbbells Only (I)

Mon, Wed and Fri or Tues, Thurs and Sat

Exercise	Sets	Reps
Stretching and Warm-Up		
1. Dumbbell Bench Press	1–3 ×	10–15
2. Flat Bench Flye	1–3 ×	12–20
3. Seated Dumbbell Press	1–3 ×	10–15
4. Lateral Raise	1–3 ×	12–20
5. Bent-Over Raise	1–3 ×	12–20
6. One-Arm Dumbbell Row	1–3 ×	10–15
7. Dumbbell Curl	1–3 ×	10–15
8. One-Arm Tricep Extension	1–3 ×	10–15
9. Shrug	1–2 ×	10–20
10. Lunge with Dumbbells	1–3 ×	10–20
11. Squat with Dumbbells	1–3 ×	10–20
12. Dumbbell Standing Calf Raise	1–3 ×	20
13. Side Bend with Dumbbell	1–3 ×	10–50
14. Crunch (Dumbbell Optional)	1–3 ×	10–50
Aerobics Optional		

INTERMEDIATE WEIGHT-TRAINING WORKOUTS

Intermediate Weight-Training Workout (A)
This is a muscle-building, bodybuilding workout for maximum gains. I recommend that you do the beginning workouts for up to six months or even a year before attempting this workout.

Mon and Fri

Exercise	Sets	Reps
Stretching and Warm-Up		
1. Bench Press	1 ×	15
	1 ×	10
	1 ×	8
	3 ×	6– 8
	1 ×	10–15
2. Incline Dumbbell Press	1 ×	15
	4 ×	6– 8
3. Flat Bench Dumbbell Press	3 ×	8–12
4. Behind-the-Neck Press	4 ×	8
5. Dip	3 ×	maximum
6. Tricep Push-Down	4 ×	8–12
7. Lateral Raise	3 ×	10–15
8. Shrug	2 ×	15–20
9. Crunch	3 ×	10–50

Tues and Sat

Exercise	Sets	Reps
Stretching and Warm-Up		
1. Squat	1 ×	20
	1 ×	15
	1 ×	10
	4 ×	8
2. Leg Press	1 ×	15
	1 ×	10
	3 ×	8
3. Leg Extension	4–5 ×	10–15
4. Leg Curl	4–5 ×	10–15
5. Donkey Raise	3 ×	10–30
6. Leg Raise	2–3 ×	10–50

Wed
Rest.

Thurs

Exercise	Sets		Reps
Stretching and Warm-Up			
1. Wide-Grip Pull-Up	4	×	maximum
2. Lat Pull-Down to Front	4	×	8–10
3. Lat Pull-Down to Rear	4	×	8–10
4. Long Pulley Row	3	×	8–10
5. Flat-Back Deadlift	3	×	8–10
6. Barbell Curl	4	×	10–15
7. Dumbbell Curl	3	×	10–15
8. Reverse Curl	3	×	10–20
9. Crunch	2–3	×	10–50

Sun
Rest.

Intermediate Weight-Training Workout (B)

As above, this is another size-building bodybuilding, not to be attempted until after six months to a year of regular training.

Mon and Fri

Exercise	Sets		Reps
Stretching and Warm-Up			
1. Bench Press	1	×	15
	1	×	10
	3	×	6– 8
	3	×	4– 6
	1	×	10–15
2. Incline Press	4	×	6–10
3. Seated Dumbbell Press	4	×	8–10
4. Behind-the-Neck Press	4	×	8–12
5. Dip	4	×	maximum
6. Tricep Push-Down	4	×	10–12

Tues and Sat

Exercise	Sets		Reps
Stretching and Warm-Up			
1.Squat	1	×	20
	1	×	15
	1	×	8
	4	×	6–10
2. Power Clean	1	×	8
	1	×	6
	3	×	3
3. Leg Extension	4	×	8–12

4. Leg Curl	4	×	8–12
5. Standing Calf Raise	4	×	8–12
6. Hyperextension	3	×	10–20

Wed
Rest.

Thurs and Sun

Exercise	Sets		Reps
Stretching and Warm-Up			
1. Bent-Over Row	5	×	8–10
2. Long Pulley Row	4	×	8–12
3. Lat Pull-Down to Front	4	×	8–12
4. Shrug	3	×	12–15
5. EZ-Bar Curl	4	×	12
6. Dumbbell Curl	4	×	12
7. Incline Sit-Up	2–4	×	10–30
8. Reverse Curl	2–4	×	10–20

Intermediate Weight-Training Workout (C)

This workout involves the use of alternating supersets and split routines (dividing your workouts by body parts on different days). You can do the same split workout exercises without using supersets, of course. You can do chest, shoulders, back and arms on Monday and Wednesday, or Monday and Thursday, and do your thighs, hamstrings, calves and abdominals on opposite days (Wednesday and Saturday or Tuesday and Friday). Here is the interesting superset split routine:

Mon, Wed and Fri
Pectorals, Deltoids, Triceps and Abdominals

Exercise	Sets		Reps
Stretching and Warm-Up			
1. Incline Dumbbell Press alternated with:	3–5	×	10–15
2. Incline Flye	3–5	×	10–15
3. Seated Dumbbell Press alternated with:	3–5	×	10–15
4. Lateral Raise	3–5	×	10–15
5. Tricep Push-Down alternated with:	3–5	×	10–15
6. Lying Tricep Extension	3–5	×	10–15
7. Crunch alternated with:	3–5	×	10–50

8. Leg Raise	3–5 × 10–30

Tues and Sat
Thighs, Hamstrings, Calves, Back and Biceps

Exercise	Sets	Reps
Stretching and Warm-Up		
1. Squats	3–5 ×	8–15
alternated with:		
2. Leg Extension	3–5 ×	10–15
alternated with:		
3. Leg Curl	3–5 ×	10–15
4. Donkey Raise	3–5 ×	10–30
alternated with:		
5. Seated Calf Raise	3–5 ×	10–30

I recommend that you do aerobics either on your weight-training workout days or on alternate days.

Intermediate Weight-Training Workout (D)

Mon and Thurs

Exercise	Sets	Reps
Stretching and Warm-Up		
1. Crunch	2–4 ×	10–50
2. Leg Raise	2–4 ×	10–30
3. Squat	3–4 ×	10–15
4. Hack Squat	3–4 ×	12–20
5. Flat-Back Deadlift	2–4 ×	10–12
6. Leg Curl	3–4 ×	12–20
7. Leg Extension	3–4 ×	12–15
8. Dip	2–4 ×	maximum
9. Tricep Push-Down	2–4 ×	12–15
10. Scott Curl	2–4 ×	10–12
11. Dumbbell Curl	2–4 ×	10–15
12. Reverse Curl	2–3 ×	10–20
13. Donkey Raise	2–3 ×	10–30

Tues and Fri

Exercise	Sets	Reps
Stretching and Warm-Up		
1. Lat Machine Crunch	2–4 ×	10–30
2. Lean-Back Twist	2–4 ×	10–30
3. Wide-Grip Pull-Up	2–4 ×	maximum
4. Lat Pull-Down to Rear	2–4 ×	10–15
5. Incline Dumbbell Press	2–4 ×	8–12
6. Incline Flye	2–4 ×	10–15
7. Seated Dumbbell Press	2–4 ×	8–12

8. Lateral Raise	2–4 × 10–15
9. Bent-Over Raise	2–4 × 10–15
10. Shrug	1–3 × 10–20
11. Regular Wrist Curl	1–3 × 10–30
12. Reverse Wrist Curl	1–3 × 10–30

MORE SPLIT ROUTINES

Some split routines are part of intermediate workouts, but some complex split routines are better left to advanced trainees. For instance, a six-day split or a double split (training twice a day) are very advanced workouts and you shouldn't attempt them if you haven't been training for well over a year, and, in the case of the double split, many weight trainees should never do them.

I consider the following split routines part of intermediate training. On most split systems, you train by body parts, that is, you train different body parts on different days. The original idea of the split system was to train your upper body one day and your lower body the next, but it quickly evolved beyond that simplistic approach.

Here are some popular muscle groupings on an intermediate split system known as the three-day-on, one-day-off system. It is very common and it's logical because you still work upper-body exercises alternating with lower-body exercises, the fundamental tenet of the split system.

Mon: Chest, Shoulders and Triceps.
Tues: Thighs, Hamstrings, Calves and Abdominals.
Wed: Back and Arms.
Thurs: Rest.
Fri: Chest, Shoulders and Triceps.
Sat: Thighs, Hamstrings, Calves and Abdominals.
Sun: Back and Arms.

Intermediate Weight-Training Workout (E)

Mon and Fri

Exercise	Sets	Reps
Stretching and Warm-Up		
1. Bench Press	1 ×	15
	1 ×	10
	5 ×	8–10

Exercise	Sets	Reps
2. Incline Dumbbell Press	1 × 15
	4 × 10
3. Behind-the-Neck Press	1 × 15
	4 × 8–10
4. Lateral Raise	4 × 10–15
5. Dip	4 × maximum
6. Tricep Push-Down	3 × 8–10
7. Crunch	4 × 10–50

Tues and Sat

Exercise	Sets	Reps
Stretching and Warm-Up		
1. Squat	1 × 20
	1 × 15
	3 × 10
	3 × 6–8

On your squats, you should progressively increase your weight as you decrease your repetitions.

Exercise	Sets	Reps
2. Leg Press	5 × 10–15
3. Leg Extension	5 × 10–15
4. Leg Curl	5 × 12–15
5. Donkey Raise	4 × 15–30

Wed and Sun

Exercise	Sets	Reps
Stretching and Warm-Up		
1. Wide-Grip Pull-Up	4 × maximum
2. Bent-Over Row	4 × 10–15
3. Lat Pull-Down to Front	5 × 8–12
4. Long Pulley Row	4 × 10–12
5. Flat-Back Deadlift	3 × 8–12
6. Barbell Curl	3 × 10–12
7. Dumbbell Curl	3 × 10–12
8. Leg Raise	3 × 10–30

Thurs
Rest.

Another popular five-day split body-part division is as follows:

Mon: Abdominals, Chest, Upper Back and Calves.
Tues: Thighs, Lower Back and Forearms.
Wed: Shoulders, Arms, Calves and Abdominals.
Thurs: Rest.
Fri: Abdominals, Chest, Upper Back and Calves.
Sat: Thighs, Lower Back and Forearms.
Sun: Shoulders, Arms, Calves and Abdominals.

Intermediate Weight-Training Workout (F)

Mon and Fri

Exercise	Sets	Reps
Stretching and Warm-Up		
1. Crunch	2–5 × 10–30
2. Leg Raise	3 × 10–30
3. Incline Dumbbell Press	3–5 × 10–15
4. Flat Bench Dumbbell Press	3–5 × 10–12
5. Dip	2 × maximum
6. Wide-Grip Pull-Up	3 × maximum
7. Lat Pull-Down to the Front	3–5 × 10–15
8. Long Pulley Row	3–5 × 10–15
9. Donkey Raise	3 × 10–30

Tues and Sat

Exercise	Sets	Reps
Stretching and Warm-Up		
1. Squat	5 × 8–15
2. Smith Rack Squat	3 × 10–20
3. Hack Squat	3 × 10–15
4. Leg Press	3 × 10–20
5. Leg Extension	3 × 15
6. Standing Leg Curl	3 × 15
7. Hyperextension	2 × 15–20
8. Reverse Curl	2 × 20–30

Wed

Exercise	Sets	Reps
Stretching and Warm-Up		
1. Incline Sit-Up	4 × 10–50
2. Side Sit-Up	4 × 10–50
3. Behind-the-Neck Press	4 × 8–15
4. Seated Dumbbell Press	4 × 10–15
5. Lateral Raise	3 × 15–20
6. Dumbbell Press	3 × 12–15
7. EZ-Bar Curl	3 × 12–15
8. Tricep Push-Down	3 × 12–15

9. Lying Tricep Extension	3 ×	12–15
10. Seated Calf Raise	3 ×	15–20

Thurs: Rest.
Fri: Repeat Mon
Sat: Repeat Tues
Sun: Rest.

ADVANCED WEIGHT-TRAINING WORKOUTS

The six-day split is an advanced workout. I really recommend against using such arduous workouts unless you have been training hard and regularly for at least a year and only if you have a lot of time, energy and motivation to succeed. The six-day split can be designed like the five-day split with a couple of exceptions: You now train an extra day and you'll train your back and biceps another day. Critical to any one training on a six-day split is recovery. *No routine is good if you can't recover!* Don't be afraid to rush to a hard, more complicated routine. Whatever works best *is* best!

Here's a simple six-day split:

Mon and Thurs: Chest, Back and Abdominals.
Tues and Sat: Thighs, Biceps and Abdominals.
Wed and Sun: Shoulders, Triceps and Calves.

Advanced Weight-Training Workout (A)

Mon and Thurs

Exercise	Sets	Reps
Stretching and Warm-Up		
1. Incline Press	5 ×	8–12
2. Flat Bench Dumbbell Press	5 ×	8–12
3. Incline Flye	4 ×	10–15
4. Dip	4 ×	maximum
5. Lat Pull-Down to the Front	5 ×	8–15
6. Long Pulley Row	5 ×	8–15
7. One-Arm Row	5 ×	12–15
8. Dumbbell Pullover	3 ×	10–20
9. Lat Machine Crunch	3 ×	10–20

Tues and Sat

Exercise	Sets	Reps
Stretching and Warm-Up		
1. Squat	6 ×	8–15
2. Hack Squat	5 ×	10–15
3. Leg Press	5 ×	10–15
4. Leg Extension	5 ×	10–15
5. Leg Curl	5 ×	10–20
6. Standing Calf Raise	4 ×	10–30
7. Seated Calf Raise	3 ×	10–30
8. Scott Curl	5 ×	10
9. EZ-Bar Curl	5 ×	10
10. Crunch	4 ×	10–50
11. Advanced Leg Raise	4 ×	10–25

Wed and Sun

Exercise	Sets	Reps
Stretching and Warm-Up		
1. Seated Behind-the-Head Press	6 ×	10–15
2. Front Dumbbell Raise	5 ×	10–15
3. Lateral Raise	5 ×	10–15
4. Bent-Over Raise	5 ×	15–20
5. Dip	4 ×	maximum
6. Tricep Push-Down	4 ×	12–15
7. Lying Tricep Extension	4 ×	12–15
8. Donkey Raise	4 ×	10–30
9. Seated Calf Raise	4 ×	10–30

THE DOUBLE SPLIT

Here is a size-building workout, using a double split. The double split is the most advanced workout.

Mon A.M.: Chest and Abdominals.
Mon P.M.: Back and Calves.
Tues A.M.: Shoulders and Triceps.
Tues P.M.: Biceps, Abdominals and Forearms.
Wed A.M.: Hamstrings and Calves.
Wed P.M.: Thighs and Abdominals.
Thurs: Rest.
Fri: Repeat Mon.
Sat: Repeat Tues.
Sun: Repeat Wed.

Advanced Weight-Training Workout (B)

Mon A.M.

Exercise	Sets		Reps
Stretching and Warm-Up			
1. Incline Press	6	×	8–12
2. Bench Press	5	×	10–15
3. Dumbbell Bench Press	5	×	8–12
4. Incline Flye	3	×	15
5. Dip	3	×	maximum
6. Incline Sit-Up	3	×	20–30
7. Crunch	3	×	20–50

Mon P.M.

Exercise	Sets		Reps
Stretching and Warm-Up			
1. Wide-Grip Pull-Up	6	×	maximum
2. Lat Pull-Down to the Front	6	×	10–12
3. Bent-Over Row	5	×	8–15
4. Long Pulley Row	5	×	10–12
5. Flat-Back Deadlift	4	×	8–15
6. Donkey Raise	5	×	15
7. Standing Calf Raise	5	×	15

Tues A.M.

Exercise	Sets		Reps
Stretching and Warm-Up			
1. Behind-the-Neck Press	2	×	10–12
	2	×	8–10
	2	×	6–8
	1	×	15
2. Seated Dumbbell Press	4	×	8–12
3. Lateral Raise	4	×	8–12
4. Bent-Over Raise	4	×	10–15
5. Tricep Push-Down	5	×	10–15
6. Tricep Kickback	4	×	10–12
7. Dip	3	×	maximum

Tues P.M.

Exercise	Sets		Reps
Stretching and Warm-Up			
1. Curl	5	×	10–15
2. Alternate Dumbbell Curl	5	×	10–15
3. Scott Curl	3	×	10–15
4. Concentration Curl	3	×	15
5. Incline Sit-Up	5	×	25–50
6. Crunch	4	×	25–50
7. Side Sit-Up	3	×	25–50
8. Leg Raise	3	×	25–35
9. Reverse Curl	3	×	10–20
10. Regular Wrist Curl	2	×	20–30
11. Reverse Wrist Curl	2	×	20–30

Wed A.M.

Exercise	Sets		Reps
Stretching and Warm-Up			
1. Leg Curl	5	×	10–20
2. Standing Leg Curl	5	×	10–20
3. Flat-Back Deadlift	4	×	10
4. Hyperextension	3	×	20
5. Donkey Raise	5	×	20–30
6. Standing Calf Raise	5	×	12–20
7. Seated Calf Raise	4	×	20–30

Wed P.M.

Exercise	Sets		Reps
Stretching and Warm-Up			
1. Squat	5	×	8–15
2. Leg Press	5	×	10–20
3. Hack Squat	4	×	10–15
4. Leg Extension	5	×	10–20
5. Cory Lunge	5	×	10–20
6. Step-Up	4	×	20–25

Thurs: Rest.
Fri: Repeat Mon.
Sat: Repeat Tues.
Sun: Repeat Wed.

MY FAVORITE ADVANCED WORKOUT FOR EACH BODY PART

Chest

Exercise	Sets		Reps
Stretching and Warm-Up			
1. Incline Dumbbell Press	6–8	×	10–15
2. Flat Bench Dumbbell Press	5–6	×	10–15
3. Pec-Deck Flye	4–5	×	15–20
4. Bench Press	4–5	×	10–15
5. Cable Crossover	3–4	×	12–20

Abdominals

Exercise	Sets		Reps
Stretching and Warm-Up			
1. Incline Sit-Up	2–4	×	20–50
2. Lat Machine Crunch	2–4	×	10–30
3. Leg Raise	3	×	20–50
4. Lean-Back Twist	3	×	20–50
5. Side Sit-Up	3	×	20–50
6. Crunch	3	×	30–50

Back

Exercise	Sets		Reps
Stretching and Warm-Up			
1. Wide-Grip Pull-Up	5–6	×	10–20
2. Lat Pull-Down to the Front	4–5	×	10–15
3. Long Pulley Row	4–5	×	10–20
4. One-Arm Row	4–5	×	10–15
5. Lat Pull-Down to the Rear	4–5	×	10–15
6. Flat-Back Deadlift	4	×	12

Legs (Thighs, Hamstrings and Calves)

Exercise	Sets		Reps
Stretching and Warm-Up			
1. Squat	6–8	×	10–20
2. Leg Press	4–5	×	10–20
3. Smith Squat	4–5	×	10–15
4. Hack Squat	3–4	×	10–15
5. Leg Extension	4–6	×	10–20
6. Leg Curl	4–6	×	10–20
7. Standing Leg Curl	3–4	×	12–15
8. Cory Lunge	2–3	×	12–20
9. Donkey Raise	3–5	×	10–20
10. Standing Calf Raise	2–3	×	10–20
11. Seated Calf Raise	2–3	×	15–20

Shoulders

Exercise	Sets		Reps
Stretching and Warm-Up			
1. Seated Dumbbell Press	4–6	×	10–15
2. Behind-the-Neck Press	4–6	×	10–15
3. Lateral Raise	5–6	×	15–20
4. Bent-Over Raise	5–6	×	15–20
5. Cable Lateral Raise	4–5	×	15–20
6. Shrug	3	×	15–20

Arms (Biceps, Triceps and Forearms)

Exercise	Sets		Reps
Stretching and Warm-Up			
1. Curl	4–6	×	10–20
2. Alternate Dumbbell Curl	4–6	×	10–15
3. Scott Curl	4–6	×	10–15
4. Concentration Curl	3–4	×	15–20
5. Tricep Push-Down	4–6	×	10–20
6. Lying Tricep Push-Down	4–6	×	10–20
7. Tricep Kickback	3–4	×	15–20
8. Regular Wrist Curl	2–3	×	20–30
9. Reverse Wrist Curl	2–3	×	20–30

HOW I GROUP MY BODY PARTS

Mon: Chest, Back and Biceps.
Tues: Thighs, Hamstrings, Lower Back and Calves.
Wed: Shoulders, Triceps and Abdominals.
Thurs: Rest.
Fri: Repeat Mon.
Sat: Repeat Tues.
Sun. Repeat Wed.

AN EXAMPLE OF PUTTING IT TOGETHER: AEROBICS, WEIGHT TRAINING AND CROSS TRAINING

This program is designed for someone with creeping middle-age spread who wants to build up lower body muscle, increase cardiovascular efficiency and lose body fat, with an emphasis on legs. It is an eight-week program to build up to a consistent exercise level.

Week One

Begin with a complete physical, including an exercise stress test. Each day do 10 minutes of easy stretching. Each day walk one mile over flat terrain. On Monday and Thursday, weight train with a program of 10 basic exercises, six for your lower body and four for your upper body. Do one set of 15–20 reps of each exercise.

Week Two

Daily 10-minute stretch. Walk 1.5 miles a day. Weight train three alternate days a week. Do 10 exercises, two sets of 15 reps each.

Weeks Three and Four

Daily 10-minute stretch. Walk two miles a day, three days a week. Weight train three alternate days a week. Do 10 exercises, two sets of 10–15 reps each. Play tennis, swim or bike ride two days a week for 20–30-minute sessions. With your abdominal exercises, do 20–50 reps.

Weeks Five and Six

Daily 10-minute stretch. Walk two miles a day, three days a week, but include some hills. Weight train three alternating days a week. Do 10 exercises, but with three sets of 10–12 reps each. Continue to do 20–50 reps with abdominal work. Play tennis, swim or bike ride two days a week, 30–40-minute sessions.

Weeks Seven through Ten

Daily 10-minute stretch. Walk two miles a day, four days a week, including hills. Weight train three alternating days a week. Do 12 exercises, three sets of 10–12 each. Any additional exercises should be lower-body exercises. Play 30–60 minutes of tennis, swim or ride a bike three days a week for 40–60 minutes.

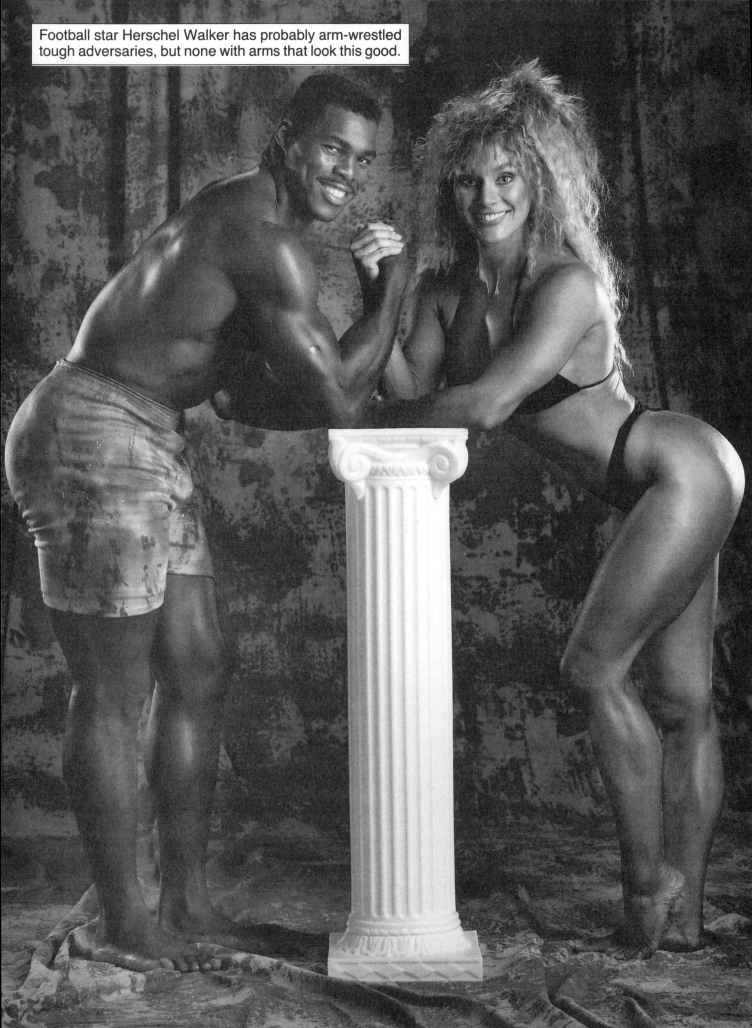

Football star Herschel Walker has probably arm-wrestled tough adversaries, but none with arms that look this good.

8

WORKOUTS FOR YOUR SPORT OR SPECIAL CONDITION

Archery
Two workouts a week.
Workout time: 40 minutes.
Rest between sets: 45 seconds.

Exercise	Sets	Reps
Warm-Up/Stretching		
1. One-Arm Dumbbell Row	3 ×	12
2. Long Pulley Row	3 ×	12
3. Lat Pull-Down to Front	2 ×	12
4. Dumbbell Press	3 ×	15
5. Bent-Over Raise	3 ×	15
6. Tricep Push-Down	2 ×	12
7. Side Sit-Up	3 ×	20–50
8. Crunch	3 ×	20–50
9. Hyperextension	2 ×	20
Cool Down		

Note: Practice and skill work 4–5 days a week.

Auto Racing
Two workouts a week.
Workout time: 40 minutes.
Rest between sets: 45 seconds.

Exercise	Sets	Reps
Warm-Up/Stretching		
1. Bench Press	3 ×	15
2. Dumbbell Press	3 ×	15
3. Lat Pull-Down to Front	2 ×	12
4. Reverse Curl	2 ×	20
5. Barbell Curl	2 ×	12
6. Tricep Push-Down	2 ×	12
7. Side Sit-Up	2 ×	20–50
8. Crunch	2 ×	20–50
9. Hyperextension	2 ×	20
Cool Down		

Note: 15 minutes of aerobics and practice and skill work 4–5 days a week.

Badminton
Two workouts a week.
Workout time: 35 minutes.
Rest between sets: 30 seconds.

Exercise	Sets	Reps
Warm-Up/Stretching		
1. Dumbbell Pull-Over	3 × 10	
2. Lat Pull-Down to Front	3 × 10	
3. Lat Machine Crunch	3 × 20–50	
4. Tricep Push-Down	2 × 12	
5. Dumbbell Press	3 × 15	
6. Flat Bench Flye	2 × 15	
7. Regular Wrist Curl	2 × 20	
8. Reverse Wrist Curl	2 × 20	
9. Leg Extension	2 × 15	
10. Leg Curl	2 × 15	
Cool Down		

Note: Work out in a circuit; 20 minutes of daily aerobics; tennis and basketball 4–6 times a week.

Baseball
Three workouts a week.
Workout time: 60 minutes.
Rest between sets: 1 minute.

Exercise	Sets	Reps
Warm-Up/Stretching		
1. Dumbbell Press	3 × 12	
2. Lateral Raise	3 × 10	
3. Incline Flye	2 × 15	
4. Lat Pull-Down to Front	3 × 15	
5. Tricep Push-Down	3 × 12	
6. Dumbbell Curl	3 × 12	
7. Reverse Curl	2 × 15	
8. Regular Wrist Curl	2 × 25	
9. Reverse Wrist Curl	2 × 25	
10. Side Sit-Up	2–3 × 20–50	
11. Crunch	2–3 × 20–50	
12. Hyperextension	2 × 15	
13. Leg Extension	2–3 × 12	
14. Leg Curl	2–3 × 12	
Cool Down		

Note: Practice and skill work 4–5 days a week.

Basketball
Three workouts a week.
Workout time: 50 minutes.
Rest between sets: 45 seconds.

Exercise	Sets	Reps
Warm-Up/Stretching		
1. Lat Pull-Down to Front	3 × 15	
2. Lat Pull-Down to Rear	3 × 15	
3. Dumbbell Press	2 × 15	
4. Incline Press	2 × 12	
5. Tricep Push-Down	2 × 12	
6. Squat	3 × 10	
7. Leg Press	3 × 10	
8. Leg Extension	3 × 12	
9. Leg Curl	3 × 12	
10. Calf Raise	2 × 20	
11. Regular Wrist Curl	3 × 20–30	
12. Crunch	3 × 20–50	
13. Hyperextension	2 × 20	
Cool Down		

Note: Train in a circuit manner; 20 minutes of sprinting, bounding and jumping, plus practice 3–4 days a week.

Bowling
Two workouts a week.
Workout time: 35 minutes.
Rest between sets: 1 minute.

Exercise	Sets	Reps
Warm-Up/Stretching		
1. Hyperextension	2 × 20	
2. Leg Extension	2 × 15	
3. Leg Curl	2 × 15	
4. Front Dumbbell Raise	2 × 12	
5. Lat Pull-Down to Front	2 × 12	
6. Barbell Curl	2 × 10	
7. Crunch	2 × 20–50	
8. Hyperextension	2 × 15	
Cool Down		

Note: Practice and skill work 4–5 days a week.

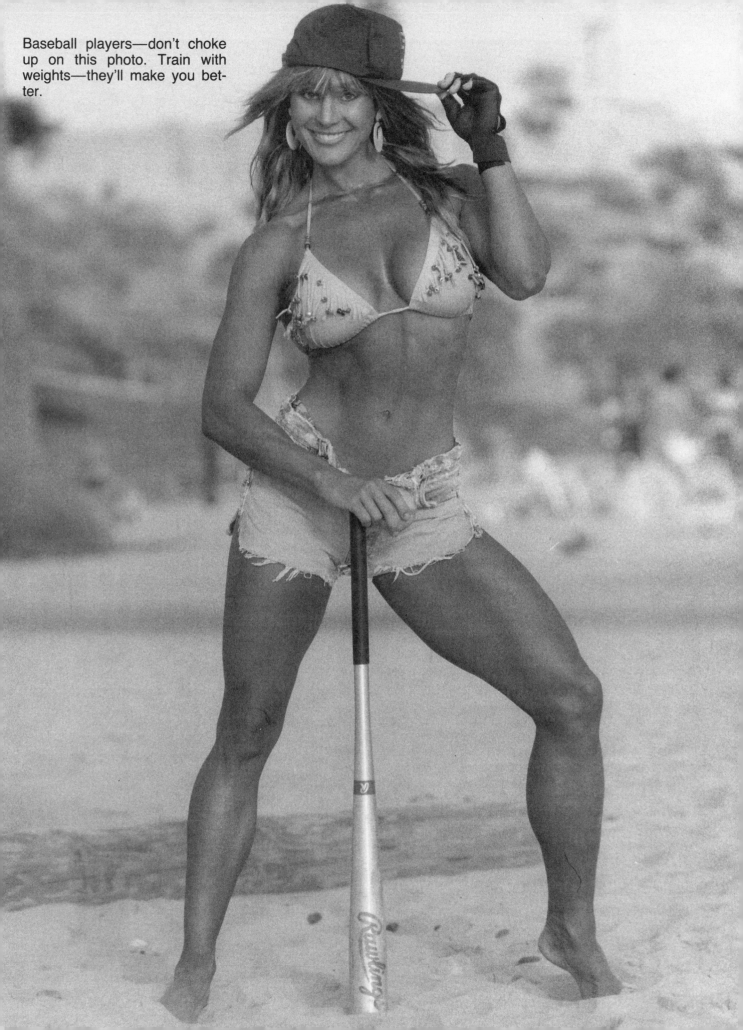

Baseball players—don't choke up on this photo. Train with weights—they'll make you better.

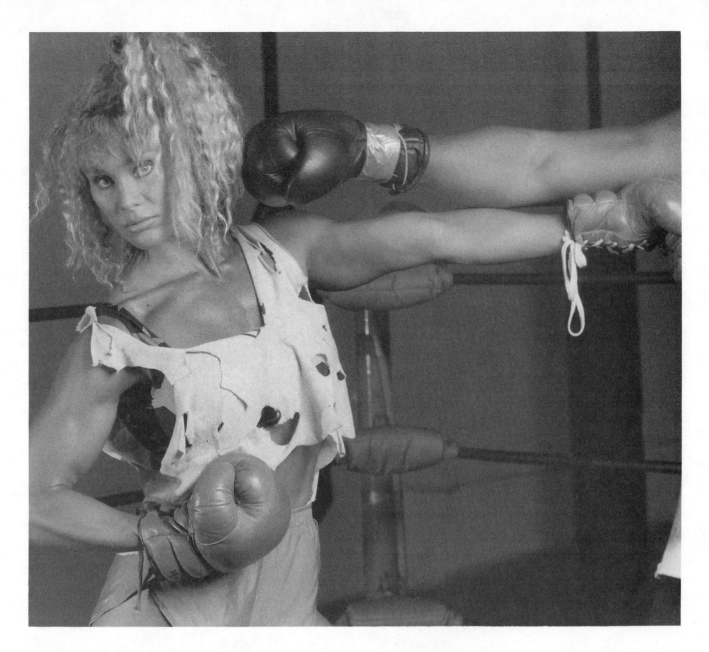

Karate, kickboxing and even the sweet science, all sharpen Cory's movie-action skills.

Boxing
Three workouts per week.
Workout time: 70 minutes.
Rest between sets: 30 seconds.

Exercise	Sets	Reps
Warm-Up/Stretching		
1. Dumbbell Press	3 ×	20
2. Lat Pull-Down to Front	3 ×	15
3. Incline Dumbbell Press	3 ×	15
4. Flat Bench Flye	2 ×	15
5. Tricep Extension	3 ×	12
6. Dumbbell Curl	3 ×	12
7. Incline Sit-Up	3–4 ×	20–50
8. Squat	4 ×	20
9. Leg Press	3 ×	15
10. Leg Extension	3 ×	15
11. Leg Curl	3 ×	15
12. Flat-Back Deadlift	3 ×	15
13. Regular Wrist Curl	3 ×	20–50
14. Standing Calf Raise	2 ×	25
15. Neck Exercise	2 ×	15 each direction

Cool Down

Note: 30 minutes of aerobics, intervals, sprints, bounding, jogging and practice and skill work, 4–6 days a week.

Crew/Canoe/Kayak/Rowing
Three workouts a week.
Workout time: 75 minutes.
Rest between sets: 30 seconds.

Exercise	Sets	Reps
Warm-Up/Stretching		
1. Hyperextension	3 ×	20
2. Long Pulley Row	3 ×	15
3. Lat Pull-Down to Front	3 ×	15
4. Pull-Up	4 ×	maximum
5. Flat-Back Deadlift	2 ×	15
6. Bent-Over Row	3 ×	15
7. Squat	5 ×	20
8. Leg Press	4 ×	20
9. Leg Extension	3 ×	20
10. Leg Curl	3 ×	20
11. Barbell Curl	3 ×	15
12. Crunch	4 ×	30–50
Cool Down		

Note: 45–60 minutes of aerobics, basketball, sprints and jogging and practice and skill work 3–5 days a week.

Cross-Country Running
Two workouts a week.
Workout time: 35 minutes.
Rest between sets: None.

Exercise	Sets	Reps
Warm-Up/Stretching		
1. Squat	1 ×	20
2. Leg Press	1 ×	20
3. Leg Extension	1 ×	20
4. Leg Curl	1 ×	20
5. Step-Up	1 ×	20
6. Crunch	1 ×	20
7. Lat Pull-Down to Front	1 ×	20
8. Dumbbell Press	1 ×	20
9. Dumbbell Curl	1 ×	20
10. Hyperextension	1 ×	20
11. Crunch	1 ×	20
Cool Down		

Note: The first six exercises are three circuits without rest between exercises. The last group of upper-body exercises are two circuits without rest between exercises; 30–60 minutes of basketball, swimming and various track drills 3–5 days a week.

Cycling
Two workouts a week.
Workout time: 50 minutes.
Rest between sets: 30 seconds.

Exercise	Sets	Reps
Warm-Up/Stretching		
1. Squat	3 ×	15
2. Leg Press	3 ×	15
3. Step-Up	3 ×	15
4. Lunge	2 ×	15
5. Leg Extension	3 ×	15
6. Leg Curl	3 ×	15
7. Power Clean	3 ×	10
8. Hyperextension	2 ×	20
9. Lat Pull-Down to Front	2 ×	15
10. Dumbbell Press	2 ×	15
11. Dumbbell Curl	2 ×	15
12. Crunch	3 ×	20–50
Cool Down		

Note: 30–60 minutes of sprints/running, 3–5 days a week.

Field Hockey
Two workouts a week.
Workout time: 45 minutes.
Rest between sets: 45–60 seconds.

Exercise	Sets	Reps
Warm-Up/Stretching		
1. Squat	3 ×	15
2. Leg Press	3 ×	15
3. Leg Extension	3 ×	15
4. Leg Curl	3 ×	15
5. Barbell Press	2 ×	15
6. Lat Pull-Down to Front	2 ×	15
7. Tricep Push-Down	2 ×	15
8. Barbell Curl	2 ×	15
9. Crunch	3 ×	20–50
Cool Down		

Note: 30 minutes of sprints, bounding, jumping or basketball 3–5 days a week.

Football (Linemen)
Three workouts a week.
Training time: 90–120 minutes.
Rest between sets: 90–120 seconds.

Exercise	Sets	Reps
Warm-Up/Stretching		
1. Bench Press	3 ×	10
	3 ×	5–6

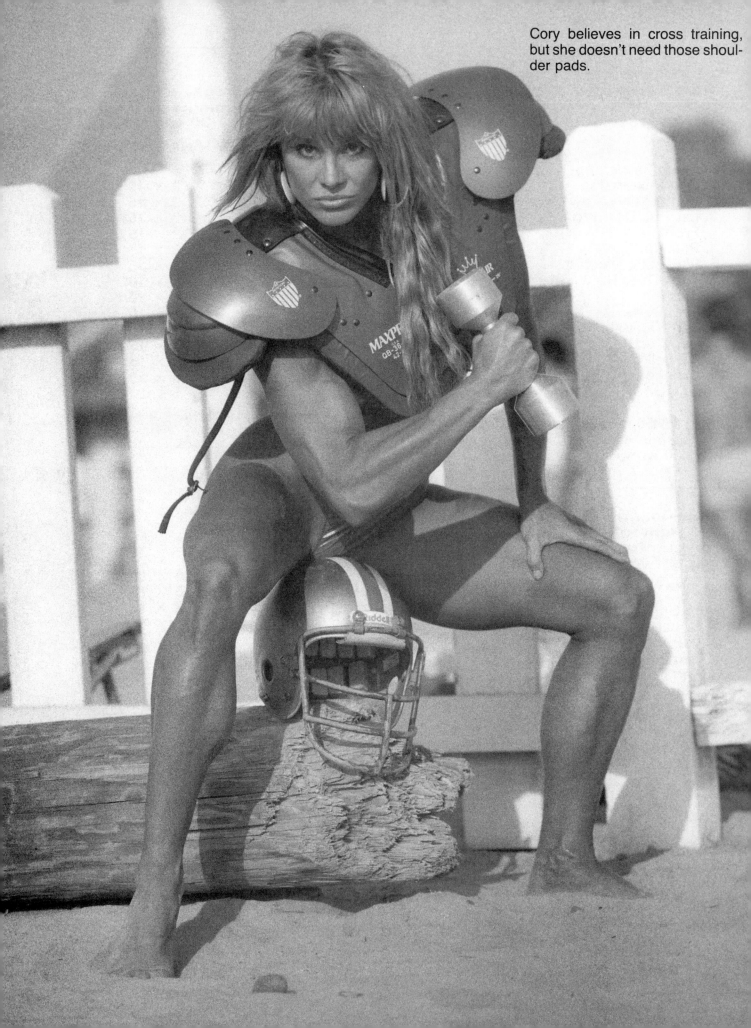

Cory believes in cross training, but she doesn't need those shoulder pads.

Exercise	Sets	Reps
2. Incline Dumbbell Press	4 ×	6– 8
3. Dumbbell Press	3 ×	8–10
4. Lat Pull-Down to Front	4 ×	6–10
5. Power Clean	4 ×	5– 6
6. Squat	3 ×	10
	3 ×	5– 6
7. Leg Press	3 ×	6– 8
8. Leg Extension	3 ×	10–12
9. Leg Curl	4 ×	10–12
10. Crunch	3 ×	20–30
11. Hyperextension	3 ×	15–20
12. Neck Exercise	2 ×	12 in all directions

Cool Down

Note: 15–25 minutes of swimming, sprints, bounding or basketball, plus practice and skill work 3–5 days a week.

Football (Linebackers and Backs)
Three workouts a week.
Workout time: 60–75 minutes.
Rest between sets: 60 seconds.

Exercise	Sets	Reps
Warm-Up/Stretching		
1. Incline Press	4 ×	8–12
2. Dumbbell Press	3 ×	8–12
3. Lat Pull-Down to Front	4 ×	8–12
4. Lat Pull-Down to Rear	3 ×	10
5. Tricep Extension	2 ×	10
6. Power Clean	4 ×	6– 8
7. Squat	4 ×	6– 8
8. Leg Extension	3 ×	12
9. Leg Curl	3 ×	12
10. Hyperextension	2 ×	20
11. Crunch	3 ×	20–50

Cool Down

Note: See previous workout recommendations.

Golf
Two workouts a week.
Workout time: 30–40 minutes.
Rest between sets: Optional.

Exercise	Sets	Reps
Warm-Up/Stretching		
1. Side Sit-Up	2 ×	20
2. Hyperextension	2 ×	20

Exercise	Sets	Reps
3. Lat Pull-Down to Front	3 ×	15
4. Squat	3 ×	15
5. Leg Extension	2 ×	20
6. Leg Curl	2 ×	20
7. Lateral Raise	2 ×	20
8. Regular Wrist Curl	2 ×	20–50
9. Reverse Wrist Curl	2 ×	20–50
10. Crunch	2 ×	20–50

Cool Down

Note: Practice and skill work 4–6 days a week.

Gymnastics
Two workouts a week.
Workout time: 55 minutes.
Rest between sets: 45–60 seconds.

Exercise	Sets	Reps
Warm-Up/Stretching		
1. Dip	3 ×	maximum
2. Dumbbell Bench Press	3 ×	12–15
3. Flat Bench Flye	3 ×	12–15
4. Tricep Push-Down	3 ×	12–15
5. Dumbbell Pull-Over	2 ×	20
6. Lat Pull-Down to Front	3 ×	12–15
7. Behind-the-Neck Press	3 ×	12
8. Leg Raise	3 ×	20–40
9. Side Sit-Up	3 ×	20–40
10. Hyperextension	3 ×	20
11. Crunch	2–3 ×	30–50

Cool Down

Note: Practice and skill work 4–6 days a week, in addition to games, sprints, jumping, swimming, bounding and basketball.

Handball
Two workouts a week.
Workout time: 35 minutes.
Rest between sets: None.

Exercise	Sets	Reps
Warm-Up/Stretching		
1. Squat	3 ×	20
2. Step-Up	3 ×	20
3. Leg Press	3 ×	20
4. Leg Extension	2 ×	15
5. Leg Curl	2 ×	15
6. Lateral Raise	2 ×	15

Exercise	Sets	Reps
7. Incline Flye	2 × 15
8. Lat Pull-Down to Front	3 × 15
9. Reverse Curl	2 × 15
10. Regular Wrist Curl	2 × 25
11. Reverse Wrist Curl	2 × 25
12. Crunch	3 × 20–50
Cool Down	

Note: 30 minutes of basketball, sprints or jogging, plus practice and skill work 3–4 days a week.

Hockey
Three workouts a week.
Workout time: 60 minutes.
Rest between sets: 30 seconds.

Exercise	*Sets*	*Reps*
Warm-Up/Stretching		
1. Squat	4 × 12–15
2. Lunge	4 × 12–20
3. Leg Extension	3 × 12
4. Leg Curl	3 × 12
5. Flat-Back Deadlift	2 × 12
6. Donkey Raise	2 × 20
7. Seated Calf Raise	2 × 20
8. Lat Pull-Down to Rear	3 × 15
9. Bench Press	3 × 15
10. Dumbbell Press	2 × 15
11. Tricep Extension	2 × 15
12. Shrug	2 × 15
13. Hyperextension	2 × 20
14. Crunch	3 × 20–50
Cool Down	

Note: 45 minutes of aerobics and practice and skill work 4–5 days a week.

Kickboxing
Workout three times a week.
Workout time: 60 minutes.
Rest between sets: 30 seconds.

Exercise	*Sets*	*Reps*
Warm-Up/Stretching		
1. Hyperextension	3 × 20
2. Leg Curl	3 × 15
3. Side Leg Pulley	3 × 10
4. Rear Leg Pulley	3 × 10
5. Squat	3 × 8–10
6. Leg Press	2 × 8–10
7. Leg Extension	2 × 8–12

Exercise	Sets	Reps
8. Dumbbell Bench Press	3 × 8–10
9. Dumbbell Press	3 × 8–12
10. Lat Pull-Down to Front	3 × 12–15
11. Leg Raise	3 × 20
12. Crunch	3 × 20–50
Cool Down	

Note: 30–45 minutes of aerobics and practice and skill work 4–5 days a week.

Lacrosse
Two workouts a week.
Workout time: 40 minutes.
Rest between sets: 30 seconds.

Exercise	*Sets*	*Reps*
Warm-Up/Stretching		
1. Squat	2 × 15
2. Leg Press	2 × 15
3. Leg Extension	2 × 15
4. Leg Curl	3 × 15
5. Hyperextension	3 × 15–20
6. Lat Pull-Down to Front	3 × 12
7. Dumbbell Press	2 × 12
8. Tricep Push-Down	2 × 12
9. Reverse Curl	2 × 15
10. Regular Wrist Curl	2 × 20–30
11. Reverse Wrist Curl	2 × 20–30
12. Crunch	2 × 20–50
Cool Down	

Note: 30–45 minutes of aerobics and practice and skill work 3–5 days a week.

Martial Arts (Judo, Karate, Kung Fu, etc.)
Three workouts a week.
Workout time: 60 minutes.
Rest between sets: 60 seconds.

Exercise	*Sets*	*Reps*
Warm-Up/Stretching		
1. Power Clean	4 × 6–8
2. Squat	4 × 8–10
3. Leg Press	3 × 12
4. Leg Curl	3 × 12
5. Leg Extension	2 × 12
6. Bench Press	3 × 8–10
7. Dumbbell Press	3 × 8–10
8. Long Pulley Row	3 × 10–12

9. Lat Pull-Down to Front — 3 × 10–12
10. Dumbbell Curl — 2 × 10
11. Tricep Kickback — 2 × 10
12. Standing Calf Raise — 2 × 15
13. Hyperextension — 2 × 20
14. Advanced Leg Raise — 2 × 15
15. Crunch — 2 × 20–50
Cool Down

Note: 30 minutes of jogging, bounding, swimming and basketball, 3–4 days a week.

Cory practices a karate side kick in preparation for her film debut in *Double Impact*.

Power Lifting
Three workouts a week.
Workout time: 90–120 minutes.
Rest between sets: 2–3 minutes.

Exercise	Sets	Reps
Warm-Up/Stretching		
1. Squat	1 ×	12
(do only 2 × 10 on	1 ×	8
your middle work-	2 ×	6
day)		
	2 ×	3
	1 ×	2
	1 ×	5
	1 ×	12
2. Deadlift	1 ×	10
(Skip on your mid-	1 ×	6
dle		
workday)	3 ×	5
3. Bench Press	1 ×	15
(2 × 10 with a	1 ×	10
close grip on		
middle day)	4 ×	6
	2 ×	3

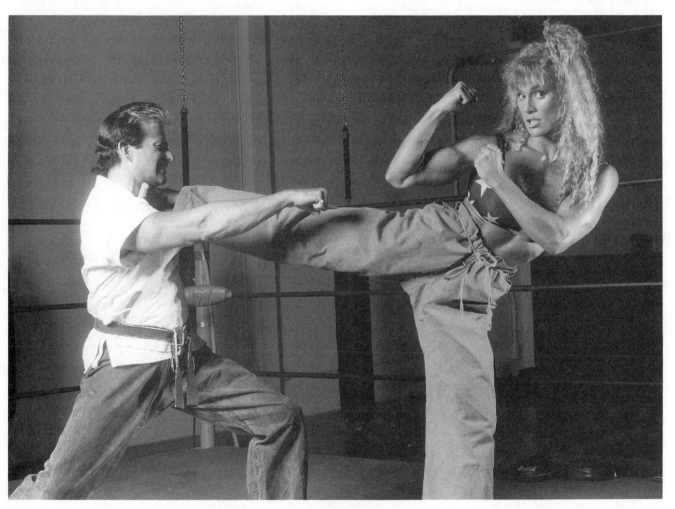

Exercise	Sets	Reps
4. Incline Dumbbell Press	3 ×	8
5. Tricep Push-Down	3 ×	6– 8
6. Dip	2 ×	maximum
7. Leg Press	2 ×	10
8. Leg Extension	2 ×	12
9. Leg Curl	4 ×	10–12
10. Hyperextension	2 ×	20
11. Crunch	3 ×	20–50

Cool Down (stretching)

Note: I recommend some daily aerobics!

Racquetball
Two workouts a week.
Workout time: 30 minutes.
Rest between sets: None.

Exercise	Sets	Reps
Warm-Up/Stretching		
1. Leg Press	2 ×	20
2. Step-Up	2 ×	15–20
3. Lunge	2 ×	15
4. Leg Extension	2 ×	15
5. Leg Curl	2 ×	15
6. Incline Flye	2 ×	20
7. Incline Press	2 ×	15
8. Tricep Push-Down	2 ×	15
9. Seated Calf Raise	2 ×	25
10. Crunch	2 ×	20–50

Cool Down

Note: 45–60 minutes of swimming, long-distance running and practice and skill work 3–4 days a week.

Rugby
Three workouts a week.
Workout time: 60–70 minutes.
Rest between sets: 45–60 seconds.

Exercise	Sets	Reps
Warm-Up/Stretching		
1. Squat	2 ×	12
	3 ×	8–10
2. Hack Squat	3 ×	12
3. Leg Press	3 ×	12
4. Leg Extension	3 ×	12
5. Leg Curl	3 ×	12
6. Barbell Press	3 ×	10
7. Bench Press	3 ×	8
8. Lat Pull-Down to Front	3 ×	10

Exercise	Sets	Reps
9. Barbell Curl	2 ×	12
10. Dip	2 ×	maximum
11. Donkey Raise	2 ×	20
12. Hyperextension	2 ×	20
13. Crunch	2 ×	20–50
14. Neck Exercise	2 ×	12 all directions

Cool Down

Note: 30 minutes of interval sprinting and jogging with skill work 3–5 days a week.

Skiing (Cross-Country)
Two workouts a week.
Workout time: 25 minutes.
Rest between sets: None.

Exercise	Sets	Reps
Warm-Up/Stretching		
1. Lunge	2 ×	25
2. Step-Up	2 ×	25
3. Squat	2 ×	25
4. Leg Press	2 ×	20
5. Leg Curl	2 ×	20
6. Leg Extension	2 ×	20
7. Seated Calf Raise	2 ×	25
8. Hyperextension	2 ×	20
9. Crunch	2 ×	20–50

Cool Down

Note: 45–60 minutes of interval sprinting, jumping, bounding and running with specific skill work 3–4 days a week.

Skiing (Downhill/Water/Jumping)
Two workouts a week.
Workout time: 30 minutes.
Rest between sets: 30 seconds.

Exercise	Sets	Reps
Warm-Up/Stretching		
1. Squat	2 ×	15
2. Leg Press	2 ×	15
3. Step-Up	2 ×	15
4. Lunge	2 ×	15
5. Leg Curl	2 ×	15
6. Leg Extension	2 ×	15
7. Donkey Raise	1 ×	20
8. Flat-Back Deadlift	1 ×	12–15
9. Hyperextension	1 ×	20
10. Crunch	1 ×	20–50
11. Lat Pull-Down to Front	1 ×	15

12. Dumbbell Press	1 × 15
13. Tricep Push-Down	1 × 15
Cool Down	

Note: 30 minutes of sprints/jogging 3–5 days a week with practice and skill work.

Soccer
Three workouts a week.
Workout time: 60 minutes.
Rest between sets: 30 seconds.

Exercise	Sets	Reps
Warm-Up/Stretching		
1. Squat	3 × 20	
2. Leg Press	3 × 20	
3. Leg Curl	3 × 20	
4. Leg Extension	3 × 20	
5. Standing Calf Raise	2 × 20	
6. Dumbbell Press	3 × 15	
7. Lat Pull-Down to Front	3 × 15	
8. Dumbbell Pull-Over	2 × 15	
9. Crunch	2 × 20–50	
10. Hyperextension	2 × 20	
Cool Down		

Note: 45–60 minutes of aerobics and practice and skill work 4–5 days a week.

Softball
Two workouts a week.
Workout time: 50 minutes.
Rest between sets: 60 seconds.

Exercise	Sets	Reps
Warm-Up/Stretching		
1. Lateral Raise	2 × 12–15	
2. Barbell Press	2 × 12–15	
3. Rear Raise	2 × 12–15	
4. Lat Pull-Down to Front	3 × 12	
5. Lat Pull-Down to Rear	3 × 12	
6. Hyperextension	2 × 20	
7. Reverse Curl	3 × 15	
8. Side Sit-Up	3 × 20–50	
9. Crunch	2 × 20–50	
10. Forward Wrist Curl	2 × 25	

| 11. Reverse Wrist Curl | 2 × 25 |
| Cool Down | |

Note: Practice and skill work 3–4 days a week.

Speed Skating
Two workouts a week.
Workout time: 60 minutes.
Rest between sets: 30–45 seconds.

Exercise	Sets	Reps
Warm-Up/Stretching		
1. Lunge	3 × 20	
2. Leg Press	3 × 20	
3. Step-Up	3 × 20	
4. Squat	3 × 20	
5. Leg Curl	3 × 20	
6. Leg Extension	3 × 20	
7. Seated Calf Raise	2 × 25	
8. Hyperextension	2 × 20	
9. Dumbbell Press	3 × 15	
10. Dumbbell Curl	2 × 20	
11. Lat Pull-Down to Front	3 × 15	
12. Crunch	2 × 20–30	
Cool Down		

Note: 45–60 minutes of sprinting, intervals, bounding and jumping plus practice and skill work 3–6 days a week.

Swimming (Diving)
Two workouts a week.
Workout time: 55 minutes.
Rest between sets: 60 seconds.

Exercise	Sets	Reps
Warm-Up/Stretching		
1. Twisting Sit-Up	3 × 20–50	
2. Flat-Back Deadlift	2 × 10	
3. Hyperextension	3 × 20	
4. Leg Raise	3 × 20–50	
5. Crunch	3 × 20–50	
6. Lat Pull-Down to Front	3 × 10–15	
7. Dumbbell Press	3 × 10–15	
8. Incline Flye	2 × 15–20	
9. Leg Extension	2 × 12	
10. Leg Curl	2 × 12	
Cool Down		

Note: 15 minutes of sprints and practice and skill work 4–6 days a week.

Swimming (Distance)
Two workouts a week.
Workout time: 30 minutes.
Rest between sets: None.

Exercise	Sets	Reps
Warm-Up/Stretching		
1. Dumbbell Pull-Over	2 ×	25
2. Lat Machine Crunch	2 ×	20–50
3. Lat Pull-Down to Front	2 ×	15–20
4. Long Pulley Row	2 ×	15–20
5. Tricep Kickback	2 ×	12–20
6. Leg Raise	2 ×	20–50
7. Hyperextension	2 ×	20
8. Leg Extension	2 ×	15
9. Leg Curl	2 ×	15
Cool Down		

Note: Work out in a circuit. Do 30 minutes of jogging with practice and skill work 4–6 days a week.

Swimming (Sprints)
Three workouts a week.
Workout time: 50 minutes.
Rest between sets: 90–120 seconds.

Exercise	Sets	Reps
Warm-Up/Stretching		
1. Power Clean	4 ×	6
2. Squat	3 ×	8–10
3. Incline Dumbbell Press	3 ×	10
4. Dumbbell Pull-Over	3 ×	12
5. Lat Pull-Down to Front	3 ×	10
6. Lat Pull-Down to Rear	3 ×	12
7. Dumbbell Press	3 ×	10
8. Leg Extension	2 ×	10
9. Leg Curl	2 ×	12
10. Leg Raise	4 ×	20–50
11. Crunch	3 ×	20–50
12. Hyperextension	2 ×	15–20
Cool Down		

Note: 15 minutes of sprints (on land!), jumping and practice and skill work 3–5 days a week.

Tennis
Two workouts a week.
Workout time: 55 minutes.
Rest between sets: 30 seconds.

Exercise	Sets	Reps
Warm-Up/Stretching		
1. Dumbbell Pull-Over	3 ×	10
2. Lat Pull-Down to Front	3 ×	10
3. Tricep Extension	3 ×	10
4. Dumbbell Press	2 ×	12
5. Leg Press	3 ×	12
6. Step-Up	3 ×	15
7. Leg Extension	3 ×	15
8. Leg Curl	3 ×	15
9. Reverse Curl	2 ×	15
10. Regular Wrist Curl	3 ×	25
11. Reverse Wrist Curl	3 ×	25
12. Crunch	2 ×	20–50
Cool Down		

Note: 35–45 minutes of swimming, basketball, handball and jogging, plus practice and skill work 3–5 days a week.

Track (Sprinters, Hurdlers and Jumpers)
Three workouts a month.
Workout time: 75 minutes.
Rest between sets: 90 seconds.

Exercise	Sets	Reps
Warm-Up/Stretching		
1. Power Clean	4 ×	6– 8
2. Squat	4 ×	6– 8
3. Flat-Back Deadlift	3 ×	8–10
4. Hyperextension	2 ×	15
5. Leg Press	3 ×	12
6. Leg Extension	3 ×	8–10
7. Leg Curl	3 ×	8–10
8. Dumbbell Press	3 ×	15
9. Lat Dumbbell to Front	3 ×	15
10. Tricep Push-Down	3 ×	15
11. Leg Raise	3 ×	20–50
12. Crunch	3 ×	20–50
Cool Down		

Note: 30 minutes of jogging, basketball or swimming, plus practice and skill work 3–5 days a week.

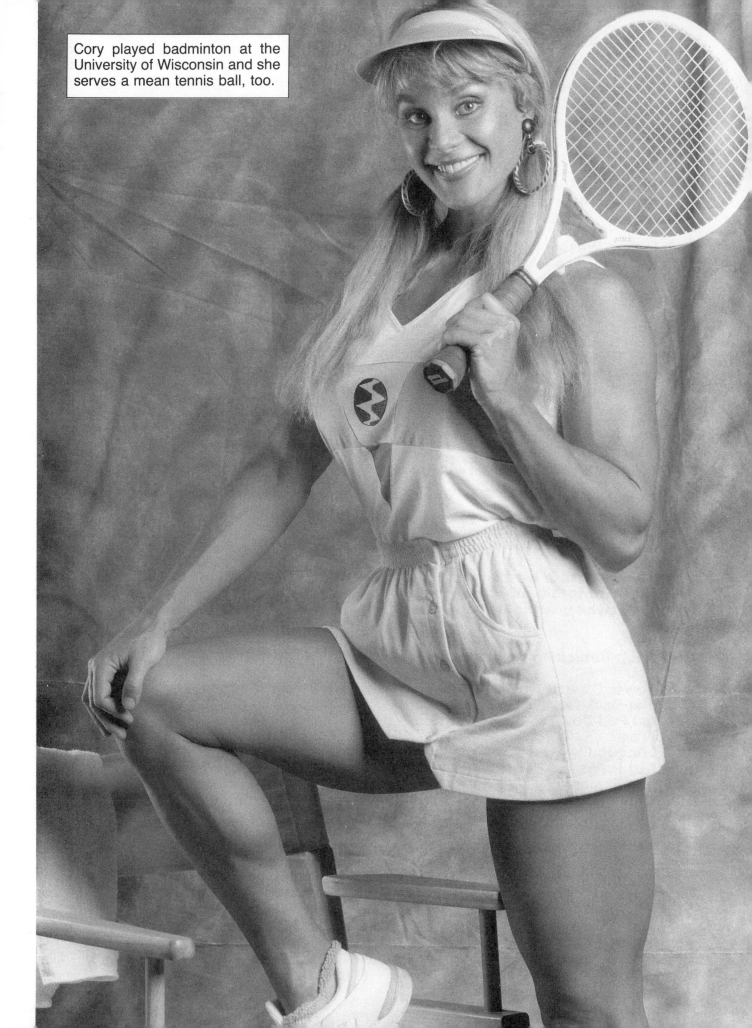

Cory played badminton at the University of Wisconsin and she serves a mean tennis ball, too.

Track (Throws)
Three workouts a week.
Workout time: 2 hours.
Rest between sets: 90–120 seconds.

Exercise	Sets		Reps
Warm-Up/Stretching			
1. Bench Press	2	×	8
	3	×	5
	1	×	3
2. Incline Press	3	×	6
3. Barbell Press	4	×	6
4. Bent-Over Row	4	×	6
5. Squat	2	×	8
	4	×	5
6. Power Clean	2	×	8
	3	×	4
7. Leg Press	3	×	8
8. Leg Extension	3	×	8
9. Leg Curl	3	×	8
10. Shrug	3	×	12
11. Crunch	2	×	20–50
Cool Down			

Note: 25-minute daily jog! Practice and skill work 3–4 days a week.

Triathlon
Two workouts a week
Workout time: 50 minutes
Rest between sets: None

Exercise	Sets		Reps
Warm-Up/Stretching			
1. Squat	3	×	15
2. Power Clean	3	×	8
3. Flat-Back Deadlift	3	×	10
4. Lat Pull-Down to Front	3	×	15
5. Long Pulley Row	3	×	15
6. Leg Press	3	×	25
7. Leg Extension	3	×	25
8. Leg Curl	3	×	25
9. Dumbbell Pull-Over	3	×	25
10. Hyperextension	3	×	25
11. Advanced Leg Raise	3	×	30–50
12. Crunch	3	×	30–50
Cool Down			

Note: Due to the severity of training, weight train only twice a week. Periodically *do not* do any of your normal training and instead go for a light jog or walk.

Volleyball
Workout two times a week.
Workout time: 50 minutes.
Rest between sets: 45 seconds.

Exercise	Sets		Reps
Warm-Up/Stretching			
1. Squat	4	×	12
2. Leg Press	3	×	12
3. Leg Curl	3	×	12
4. Leg Extension	3	×	12
5. Lat Pull-Down to Front	3	×	8–10
6. Dumbbell Press	3	×	8–10
7. Dumbbell Pull-Over	3	×	8–12
8. Tricep Extension	2	×	12–15
9. Hyperextension	2	×	20
10. Crunch	3	×	20–50
Cool Down			

Note: 30–45 minutes of daily aerobics.

Water Polo
Workout two times a week.
Workout time: 40 minutes.
Rest between sets: None.

Exercise	Sets		Reps
Warm-Up/Stretching			
1. Power Clean	3	×	10
2. Squat	3	×	12
3. Leg Press	3	×	12
4. Leg Extension	3	×	20
5. Leg Curl	3	×	20
6. Hyperextension	2	×	20
7. Dumbbell Press	3	×	20
8. Lat Machine to Front	4	×	15
9. Dip	3	×	maximum
10. Shrug	3	×	20
11. Crunch	3	×	20–50
Cool Down			

Note: 45–60 minutes of land sprints, jumping, basketball, plus practice and skill work 3–6 days a week.

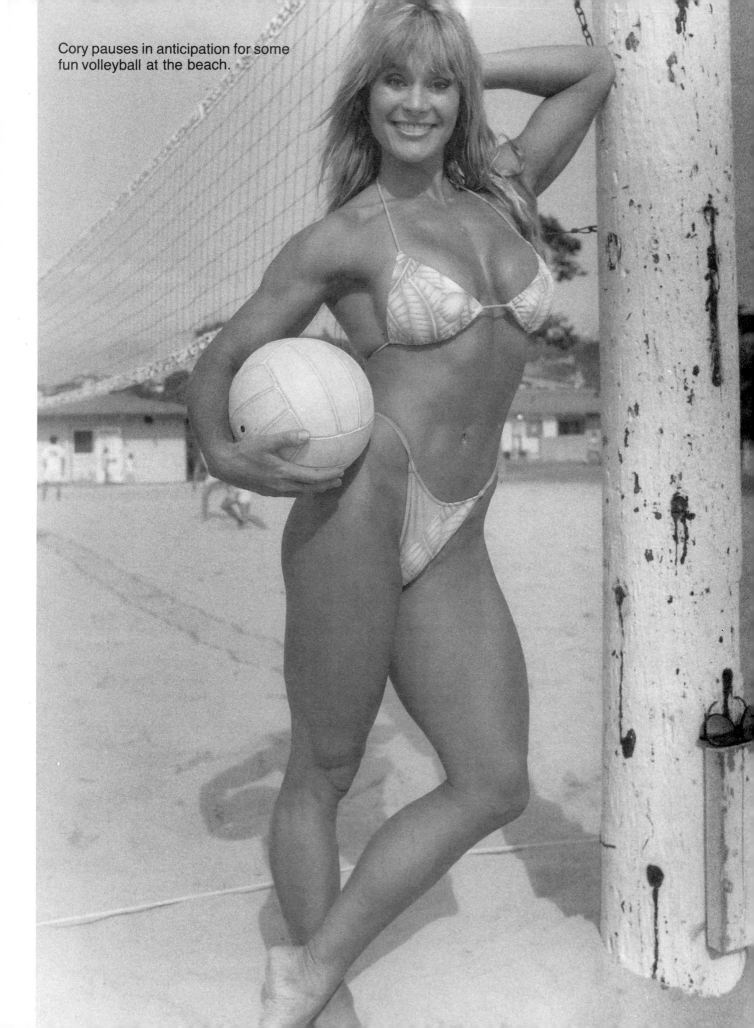

Cory pauses in anticipation for some
fun volleyball at the beach.

Weight Lifting
Work out five times a week.
Workout time: 90–120 minutes.
Rest between sets: 2–3 minutes.

Exercise	Sets	Reps
Mon and Thurs		
Warm-Up/Stretching		
1. Power Clean	2 ×	6
	5 ×	3
2. Squat	2 ×	8
	5 ×	5
3. Jerk from Stand	2 ×	6
	4 ×	3
4. Shrug	3 ×	8
5. Leg Press	3 ×	8
6. Leg Extension	3 ×	10
7. Leg Curl	3 ×	10
8. Hyperextension	3 ×	10–15
9. Crunch	3 ×	20–50
Cool Down		

Note: Do some daily aerobics.

Exercise	Sets	Reps
Wed and Sat		
Warm-Up/Stretching		
1. Clean	5 ×	3
2. Snatch	5 ×	2
3. Power Clean from Hang	4 ×	4–6
4. Power Snatch from Hang	4 ×	2–3
5. Front Squat	5 ×	6
6. Form Jerk	5 ×	2
7. Hyperextension	2 ×	20
8. Crunch	3 ×	20–30
Cool Down		

Note: Again, do some daily aerobics.

Wrestling
Work out three times a week.
Workout time: 60–75 minutes.
Rest between sets: 45–60 seconds.

Exercise	Sets	Reps
Warm-Up/Stretching		
1. Dumbbell Press	3 ×	12
2. Bench Press	3 ×	12
3. Lat Pull-Down to Front	4 ×	8–10
4. Long Pulley Row	3 ×	8–12
5. Dumbbell Row	3 ×	8–12
6. Tricep Push-Down	3 ×	8–12
7. Dip	2 ×	maximum
8. Squat	3 ×	8–10
9. Leg Extension	3 ×	8–12
10. Leg Curl	3 ×	8–12
11. Hyperextension	2 ×	20
12. Crunch	3 ×	20–50
13. Neck Work	2 ×	12 all directions
Cool Down		

Note: 30–45 minutes of sprints, jogging, swimming, and/or basketball, plus practice and skill work 3–4 days a week.

SPECIAL CONDITIONS

Knee Rehabilitation
Work out five times a week to tolerance with doctor's direction.
Workout time: 30–45 minutes.
Rest between sets: 1–2 minutes.

Exercise	Sets	Reps
Warm-Up/Stretching		
1. Leg Extension	1 ×	25
	1 ×	20
	1 ×	15
	2 ×	10
	1 ×	25
2. Leg Curl	as above	
3. Leg Press	5 ×	12
4. Half Squat	3 ×	12–20
5. Standing Calf Raise	3 ×	20

Note: Stretch daily.

Shoulder Rehabilitation
Work out five times a week to tolerance with doctor's direction.
Workout time: 35–45 minutes.
Rest between sets: 1–2 minutes.

Exercise	Sets	Reps
Warm-Up/Stretching		
1. Dumbbell Press	3 ×	15
2. Dumbbell Bench Press	3 ×	20
3. Lateral Raise	3 ×	20
4. Front Raise	3 ×	20

Exercise	Sets	Reps
5. Shrug	3 × 20
6. Dumbbell Row	3 × 15
7. Long Pulley Row	3 × 15
8. Lat Pull-Down to Front	3 × 15
9. Dumbbell Curl	2 × 15

Note: Stretch daily.

Lower-Back Rehabilitation
Four workouts a week.
Workout time: 30 minutes.
Rest between sets: 2–4 minutes.

Exercise	Sets	Reps
Warm-Up/Stretching		
1. Pelvic Tilts	3 × 15–20
2. Single Knee to Chest	2 × 20
3. Double Knee to Chest	2 × 20
4. Crunch	3 × 10–20
5. Lower-Back Extension	3 × 15–20
6. Hamstring Stretch	2 × 20
7. Leg Extension	2 × 20
8. Leg Curl	2 × 20

Note: Practice posture and mechanics! Recommended reading: *Back in Shape* by the Texas Back Institute.

Heart-Patient Rehabilitation

Follow your doctor's advice. Start with slow walking on level terrain. Go five minutes and gradually work up to an hour of walking on level terrain. With weight training, use light weights and high repetitions. Do not hold your breath or squeeze or grip hard your bars and dumbbells. Concentrate on lower-body exercises at first until your doctor agrees to upper-body exercises.

Work out three times a week.
Workout time: At your leisure.
Rest between sets: At your leisure.

Exercise	Sets	Reps
Warm-Up/Stretching		
1. Leg Extension	1 × 20
2. Leg Curl	1 × 20
3. Leg Press	1 × 20
4. Step-Up (low step)	1 × 20
5. Machine Bench Press	1 × 20
6. Lat Pull-Down to Front	1 × 15
7. Tricep Extension	1 × 20
Cool Down		

Note: Low-fat diet!!!

Workout for Kids (12–16)
Work out three times a week.
Workout time: 60 minutes.
Rest between sets: 1–2 minutes.

Exercise	Sets	Reps
Warm-Up/Stretching		
1. Pull-Up	3 × maximum
2. Push-Up	3 × maximum
3. Leg Press	3 × 12–15
4. Leg Extension	3 × 12–15
5. Leg Curl	3 × 12–15
6. Dumbbell Press	3 × 12–15
7. Dumbbell Bench Press	3 × 12–15
8. Dip	2 × maximum
9. Dumbbell Curl	2 × 12–15
10. Lat Pull-Down to Front	3 × 15
11. Hyperextension (to parallel)	2 × 20
12. Crunch	3 × 20–50
Cool Down		

Note: Do aerobics at least three times a week.

Workout for the Physically Challenged

Individuals unable to train with weights should exercise on a mat with a therapist or partner (or by yourself, if you are able to transfer to the mat and back). Balancing on all fours for strength and coordination, crawling, or partial push-ups are great muscle-toning exercises.

General Floor/Mat Exercise Program:
Work out two or three times a week.
Workout time: Optional.
Rest between sets: Optional.

Exercise	Sets	Reps
Warm-Up/Stretching *(where applicable)*		
1. Half-to-Full Crunch	1 ×	10
2. Hip Raise (with your knees to-gether, while on your back, raise your hips off the floor 10 times	1 ×	10
3. Single Bent-Leg Lift (in the position as above, try to pull your leg up as far as you can)	1 ×	10
4. Partial Push-Up (you can do these on your knees or even on your stomach)	1 ×	maximum
5. Standing Toe Raise	1 ×	10
6. Standing One-Leg Knee Lift	1 ×	10
7. Machine Bench Press	2 ×	12–15 (if applicable)
8. Lat Pull-Down to Front	2 ×	12–15 (if applicable)
9. Machine Press	2 ×	12–15 (if applicable)

Cool Down (stretching)

Thirty Something!
Work out three times a week.
Workout time: 75—90 minutes.
Rest between sets: 45—90 seconds.

Exercise	Sets	Reps
Warm-Up/Stretching		
1. Incline Dumbbell Press	3 ×	10–15
2. Incline Flye	3 ×	10–15
3. Lat Pull-Down to Front	4 ×	8–12
4. Long Pulley Row	3 ×	12–15
5. Dumbbell Press	3 ×	10–15
6. Lateral Raise	3 ×	10–15
7. Dumbbell Curl	3 ×	10–15
8. Tricep Push-Down	3 ×	10–15
9. Leg Press	3 ×	12
10. Leg Extension	3 ×	12–15
11. Leg Curl	3 ×	12–15
12. Hyperextension	1 ×	20
13. Crunch	3 ×	20–50
Cool Down		

Note: 30—60 minutes of daily aerobics.

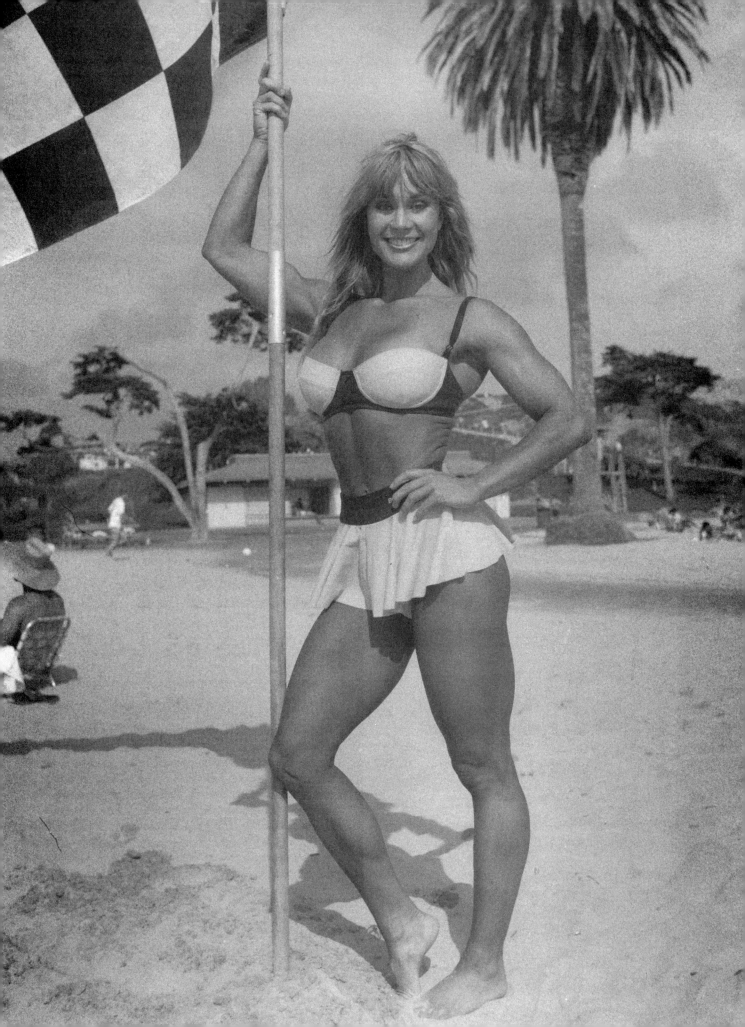

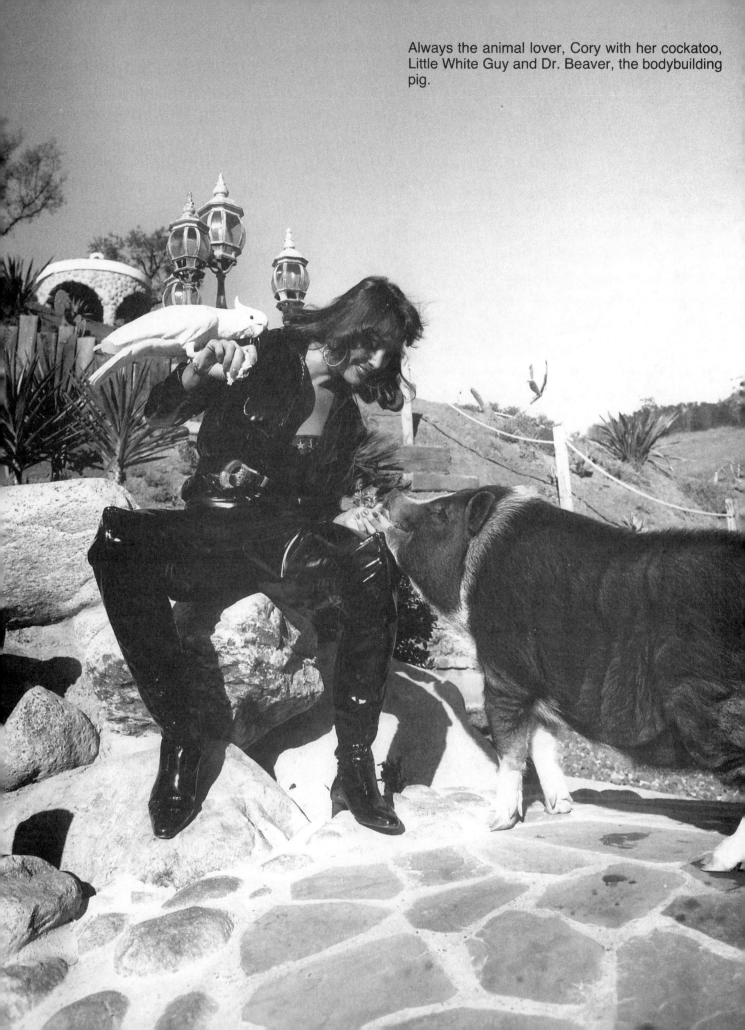

Always the animal lover, Cory with her cockatoo, Little White Guy and Dr. Beaver, the bodybuilding pig.

9

NUTRITION: YOUR FIRST STEP

It's a depressing fact that, with the standard of obesity at 20 percent more than ideal body weight, fully one out of five American women is obese. Exercise is only one-third of the battle. A fit lifestyle and good nutrition are equally important to get and stay in shape. If you eat too much and gorge yourself with fat, exercise can't make you lean or guarantee health.

If you want to lose fat weight and get in shape, get rid of the concept of diet as a deprivation and treat diet as a concept/lifestyle with calorically balanced nutrition. Eat moderately from the basic food groups with low fats, few simple sugars, low cholesterol, high carbohydrates, moderate protein, high fiber and an adequate supply of vitamins, minerals and water. This is simple in theory and should be simple to accomplish, but for most people, it's not. I'll show you how to do it!

THE BASIC FOOD GROUPS

I belong to a growing group of people who have abandoned the old four basic food groups for a revised five basic food groups. Most nutritionists now list five important food groups: fruit and vegetables (one), milk (two), grains (three), meat or protein alternatives (four) and fats (five).

The concept of four basic food groups was developed in the fifties by the U.S. Department of Agriculture. It was designed as a foundation of food types. The basic four groups have always included two servings of dairy products, two servings of meat and four servings of fruit and vegetables each day.

Depending on serving sizes, this diet does provide ample protein for most people and most of the vitamins and minerals we need (sometimes this diet is short in riboflavin or B6, zinc and magnesium, and for women, iron). But for many people, it provides too much fat and cholesterol and not enough fiber, especially considering people eat too many bad foods and indulge too often in the fast-food line.

By following a basic five, you will bring up your fiber and vitamin levels and lower your fat, provided you make some easy manipulations.

Fruit and Vegetables

It's too bad we didn't follow our mothers'

165

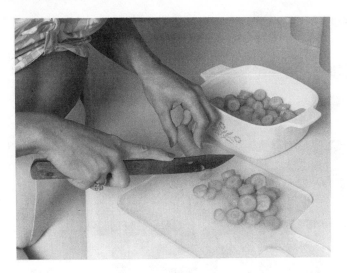

Carrots are great, high in vitamin A and low in calories.

advice about eating vegetables. As every day passes, scientists rediscover the value of vegetables and fruits, whether it's fighting some disease, like cancer or heart disease, or providing low-calorie, low-fat, low-cholesterol sources of valuable nutrients.

Without getting complex, every day you should eat at least one fruit high in vitamin C and one vegetable high in vitamin C. Doing this usually ensures an ample supply of B vitamins, too. However, you should eat a total of six servings (a serving is not all that much, about a half cup of fruit or frozen vegetables) of fruit and vegetables each day. If you choose one vitamin-C fruit and vegetable (an orange and a piece of broccoli, for example), your remaining portions should include some dark green vegetables, yellow vegetables (squash) and fruit.

Don't get hung up on counting servings. That's too boring and clinical. Instead, make an effort to eat an apple or a piece of melon, orange and banana each day and some broccoli, asparagus, carrots and/or spinach and you'll do just fine. If you drink fruit juices, try fresh, unsweetened juices. Choose fresh fruits and vegetables over canned fruits and vegetables, which usually have too much added sugar.

I'm not opposed to anyone taking a multiple vitamin-mineral tablet each day either. However, I don't think you need to swallow a medicine chest of pills if you eat correctly. Pills don't provide food energy.

Milk

Remember the good old days when you were supposed to drink whole milk and eat eggs every day? It's too bad milk has received such bad press lately. It's still an unbelievably good, calorically dense food. Many people simply don't care for its taste or that it comes from animals. I'm guilty myself: I don't drink enough of the white stuff even though I recognize its values. Some of you may have a lactose sugar intolerance, in which case you can get your nutrients from other sources or use a commercial enzyme product which will help you digest lactose.

Generally, young children, teenagers, pregnant women, the elderly and athletes should include skim or 2-percent milk in their daily diets. You only need 2–3 servings a day (one cup equals one serving). If you eat some cottage cheese, cheese or yogurt, you need even less. Low-fat milk, or preferably skim milk, provides vitamins and minerals, notably calcium, vitamin A, B complex vitamins and protein. If you can't handle milk or have a distaste for it, no problem—just make up for it elsewhere.

Meat and/or Protein Groups

Despite what some nutritionists believe, the how-much-protein-is-necessary-for-athletes debate is far from a dead issue. New research is constantly shedding light on whether hard-training athletes need more protein. In general, if you eat like an average American (too much high-fat, high-calorie food), you get enough protein.

Choose your protein from low-fat sources. A protein serving (eat three protein servings each day) is only 2–4 ounces and that's not very much considering some people eat five times that much at one meal, if they eat a full size T-bone steak and baked potato with a glass of milk!

What should be your protein sources? Fish, de-skinned chicken and turkey and water-packed tuna are great. I recommend that if you eat lean hamburger, chops or steak, do so only once every two or three weeks. Select meat as lean as possible and cut off all visible fat, and don't overeat.

All your meat should be cooked in low-fat oils and baked, broiled or poached. Don't fry meats. It doesn't take much meat

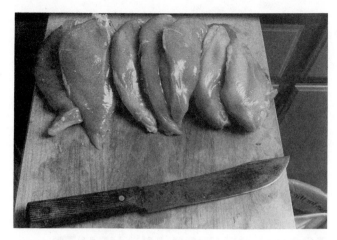
Fish and de-skinned chicken are excellent sources of dietary protein.

to satisfy your protein needs. A large tuna sandwich on whole-wheat bread without mayo, with one or two de-skinned chicken breasts and two glasses of milk over the day easily satisfies your protein needs, if you are average size.

At the risk of being controversial, in my opinion if you're a weight-trained athlete trying to lose fat and build muscle, I recommend 1.5 grams of protein per kilogram of body weight each day. This is a bit higher than some nutritionists recommend, but a lot lower than many others. If you weigh 60 kilograms (132 pounds), eat about 90 grams of first-class, low-fat protein a day. If you're inactive, one gram per kilogram of weight per day is probably enough.

Some recent scientific evidence suggests that athletes undergoing intense training go into negative nitrogen balance, losing more protein than they take in, especially if they're following low-calorie diets in an effort to lose excess fat. Needless to say, this type of nutrition isn't kosher for muscle growth.

Be that as it may, don't eat a lot more protein each day to make up for it. Eat a moderate amount of good-quality protein each day. Bodybuilders use commercial protein supplements for this purpose. These protein powders are usually an egg, soy or milk protein base and very low in fat and/or calories. The average person doesn't need protein supplements, provided they're eating normal dietary proteins. Unfortunately, fast foods, which people eat as protein sources, are devas-

tatingly high in fat, calories and sodium.

If you don't like meat or are opposed to destroying animals to supply human protein needs (I'm almost a vegetarian myself—also a Snickersetarian—and really don't eat much meat, mostly de-skinned chicken or tuna), you can still meet your protein needs, although it's a little more difficult.

Egg whites, white cheeses, skim milk, cottage cheese, fish, beans, lentils, potatoes and corn are all examples of foods that provide proteins. In my next chapter, "Nutrition: Your Final Step," I list more high-protein foods to choose from.

Grains

Once again, evidence shows that fibers and grains are not only good for your health, but may fight specific diseases, such as colon cancers. Four servings (one piece of bread is a serving, so a serving is not much) per day are recommended by most medical doctors and nutritionists.

I recommend high-fiber cereals, oatmeal, whole-grain breads, pastas and rice. Include fibers from different sources. Some time during the day, I recommend that you have a bowl of oatmeal (just like the commercial recommends), some pasta, beans, lentils, rice, fruit with skin and a couple of pieces of whole-grain bread. Eat 30 grams of fiber every day and your colon and arteries will thank you for it!

Rice is a staple of both Japanese and Chinese cultures. Rice is high in carbs, low in fat. There is little heart disease in these cultures.

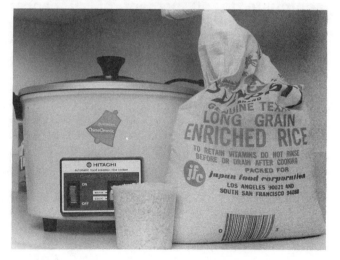

Fats

Your total daily caloric percentage of fats should be somewhere between 10–30 percent. The majority of nutritionists feel 30 percent is okay, but I think this is too high and feel that 10–20 percent is plenty. I lean toward a Pritikin eating approach for good health.

You need fats, of course. You can't survive without them. The fat tissue is complicated. The average American takes in about 40–50 percent of their total calories in the form of fat. This is a sin against your body!

Dietary fat is either saturated, mono-unsaturated or polyunsaturated. These words confuse people. Most Americans love saturated fats and of the 40–50 percent total fat we eat, most of it, usually 20–25 percent, is saturated fat. Saturated fat is usually solid at room temperature, such as butter and the fat in meat, for example.

Three fatty acids are essential for health. Your body can't produce these by itself and arachidonic, linoleic and linolenic fatty acids must be supplied from your foods. Likewise, proteins are divided into essential and nonessential amino acids and you must receive the essential amino acids from your foods. You do need some unsaturated fats, too. Basically, you need fats for insulation and energy. Fats are carriers for fat-soluble vitamins and some fat is very important to protect important body organs.

Unfortunately though, too much fat is linked to heart disease, breast cancer, diabetes and stroke. The National Cancer Institute believes that high-fat diets may contribute to 40 percent of all cancer deaths in women and 60 percent of cancers in men. High-fat diets are often linked to cancers of the uterus, ovaries, prostate, colon and breast.

A serving of fat per day is recommended. That's not much! Two to three tablespoons of vegetable oil used in cooking satisfies this! So does a pat or two of butter or a couple tablespoonfuls of salad dressing, or a couple strips of bacon. You don't need much!

For cooking oils, choose one that's low in saturated fat and higher in unsaturated fat. Remember, it's animal products and saturated fats that are high in cholesterol.

There's little cholesterol in vegetable products and none in fruit.

When cooking, use oils that are predominantly monounsaturates or polyunsaturates. This includes corn, olive, canola, sunflower and safflower oils. Don't use butter, if possible. Butter is extremely high in saturated fat and loaded to the hilt with cholesterol, about 30–33 milligrams per tablespoon.

GOOD NUTRITION AND HEALTH CONCERNS

Most of you understand that it's healthy to cut back on foods high in fat and cholesterol. However, the cholesterol subject is very confusing to many people (and to many doctors).

Cholesterol levels in humans vary from a low of about 100 milligrams per deciliter of blood to an upper level of normal set at 300 milligrams. In recent years, most doctors and those knowledgeable in the cholesterol business have said that a cholesterol level over 240 puts you "at risk" for heart disease and stroke. A second sub-group of doctors believes any level over 200 milligrams may put you at risk.

Interestingly, approximately 20 percent of all heart attacks occur in individuals with cholesterol levels under 200. This may relate to genetic factors, valve disease, muscle bridges, coronary spasms and other conditions. Or, the cholesterol issue may be even more complicated.

Although there are several types of cholesterol, doctors measure two broad classifications called HDL, high-density lipoprotein cholesterol and LDL, low-density lipoprotein cholesterol. HDL's are "good" cholesterol. LDL's are "bad" cholesterol. It's best to have a high level of HDL relative to your total cholesterol.

If you divide your total cholesterol by your HDL level, your ratio should be 3 to 1. For example, if your total cholesterol is 240 and your HDL level is 80, you are on the borderline for danger. If your total is 200 and your HDL is 100, that's much better. With a cholesterol of 160 and an HDL of 105, you have an excellent profile.

Most heart attacks take place in people with cholesterol levels between 220 and 300 milligrams. Exercise appears to elevate HDL and lower LDL, but the best way to control these values is by food. Saturated fats and cholesterol-rich foods raise your cholesterol levels.

To keep things as simple as possible, lower the fats in your diet to 10–15 percent of caloric intake. Of the fats you eat, make an effort to eliminate almost all saturated fats in lieu of polyunsaturated and monounsaturated fats. If you make a strong effort to do this *and* exercise, you should lower your cholesterol level significantly. If you have high cholesterol unaffected by exercise and diet, follow your doctor's advice on cholesterol-lowering medications.

The average American may eat 40–100 grams of saturated fat each day (against a backlog of about 80–150 grams of total fat each day, or more)! In one day, you should eat no more than 20 grams of saturated fat (if even that).

One average hamburger patty, by itself without condiments or bun, has about 15 grams of saturated fat in it! Americans might take a tip from the Chinese population. The Chinese diet is about 20 percent fat compared to our 40 percent. Their diet is particularly low in saturated fat and cholesterol and high in fiber. Heart disease is rare in China.

Remove all the chicken skin before cooking. You'll be less tempted to eat it when it's not cooked. Ugh.

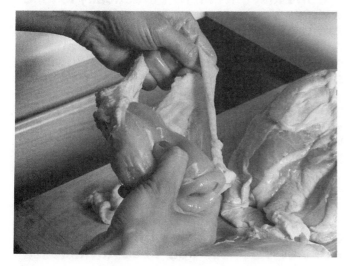

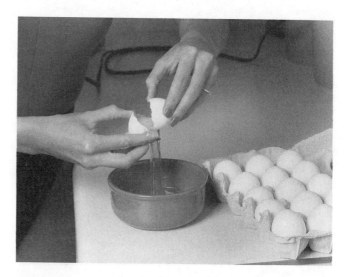

Eggs have been called the perfect food, but don't be like Rocky and eat them raw. Soft-boil them and skip the yolks.

Common Food Cholesterol Levels

Food	Satu-rated Fat (grams)	Choles-terol (milli-grams)
Beef (4 oz.)	4–5	490–550
Chicken Breast, de-skinned (4 oz.)	1–2	85–105
Egg	2–3	205–215
Liver (4 oz.)	3	500–545
McDonald's Egg McMuffin	4–5	200–230
Pork Chop (4 oz.)	4–5	103–105
Whole Milk (1 cup)	5–6	33–34
Fruit	0	0
Vegetables	0–1	0
Egg White	0	0

In my opinion, you shouldn't eat more than 300 milligrams of cholesterol a day, if at all possible. You shouldn't eat more than 20 grams of saturated fat a day, either.

WHAT ABOUT TRIGLYCERIDES?

Of that 80–150 (or more) grams of fat that most of you eat during the day, a lot of it is in the form of triglycerides. All saturated, polyunsaturated and monounsaturated fats are technically triglycerides. The balance of your dietary fat is cholesterol. Tri-

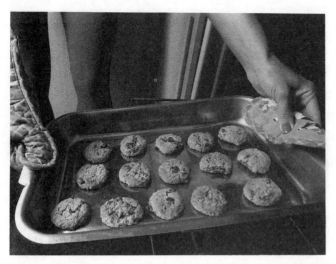

I love chocolate-chip cookies, too, but eat them only on occasion. Like most cookies, they're high in fat and sugar.

glycerides are used for energy or are stored as body fat.

Excess calories, no matter what their form, can be converted by your liver to triglycerides (fat). However, there is less likelihood of this happening if your excess calories are carbohydrates or protein, as opposed to fats.

While this might surprise you, it's easier for your body to convert excess ice-cream calories to fat than it is excess apple calories (if there is such a thing). In fact, I doubt you'll ever see someone who eats loads of fruit and vegetables and is obese. Your body just doesn't work that way.

Your doctor can tell you if your triglyceride level is too high, against a backdrop of your cholesterol level. The following foods raise your triglycerides: alcohol of all kinds, candy, cakes, pies, sweetened fruit drinks, ice cream, sweetened cereals, doughnuts and cookies.

LOSING EXCESS FAT AND LEANING OUT!

It's no secret that losing fat weight and leaning out is not easy. Many people spend their whole adult lives trying to do just that. You want to lose excess fat and then keep it off. My workouts and nutrition plans accomplish this. You should feel good about the programs you pursue to accomplish

your goals; you don't want to lose muscle while you lose fat. You have to follow a safe, realistic program.

It's possible, of course, to be thin and still too fat! You want to optimize your lean-muscle-mass-to-fat ratio. An ideal body fat percentage for adult males is around 16 percent; for women, about 20–25 percent. These figures compare to national averages of about 25–28 percent for men and 35–40 percent for women. The averages aren't healthy.

Although there are all kinds of fancy ways to measure your body fat, use some simple tests to get an idea of where you rate. With your arm straight, flex your triceps. Pinch the skin over the muscle. If you pinch more than an inch of flab, you're carrying too much fat there. Pinch the skin under the bottom of your rib cage; more than an inch there is also too much. Finally, grab the skin around your navel in the pinch test; more than two inches is too much.

Most people are quite a bit over these guidelines. They have too much fat, not enough muscle. Remember, your muscle determines your calorie needs. If you have a lot of lean mass, you'll burn more calories. If you don't have much lean mass, you can't eat as much. It's almost so simple that it's stupid.

The main reasons people have to diet all the time *are because they are too fat, and because they don't have enough muscle!* This is a universal statement, except for the chronically obese; and if most people would realize and appreciate that, there would be less problems with creeping body fat with age.

Don't just cut calories drastically to lose weight. You'll lose water and muscle instead of fat because your metabolism will read your diet as a starvation state and, in starvation, your body slows way down to save calories. Additionally, every time you yo-yo down on your calories, you lose muscle and build up certain enzymes, which tend to swell up your fat cells. So, when you go off the diet and start eating normally again, your fat cells are waiting to fill up and, thus, you blow up even fatter than you were before! Egads, such good news!

You must do a weight-training program and aerobics with any nutrition plan where you cut calories. You need to increase your muscle mass, or at least maintain it, besides burning calories and conditioning your heart. With more muscle, you can eat more, have more fun in social eating situations, maintain your energy, muscle tone and shape. Plus, you won't gain your lost fat weight back! For most of you, while losing fat is a great goal, it should *not* be your only goal.

A major goal should be increasing your lean mass. Doing so means that excess body fat will eventually take care of itself. Good health should also be your major goal and that's why learning about your foods is so important and why I spent so much time on saturated fat, triglycerides and cholesterol!

10 BASIC FOOD RULES

1. Eat less fat.
2. Eat less high-cholesterol foods.
3. Consume less foods or drinks that raise your triglycerides.
4. Eat more unrefined carbohydrates, such as fruit, rice, pasta and potatoes.
5. Eat less sugar and sodium.
6. Drink more water.
7. Eat more vegetables and fiber.
8. Weight train.
9. Do aerobics.
10. Increase your activity level.

SOME MORE FOOD GUIDELINES

1. If you're only a few pounds off your ideal weight, make a small deduction from your normal calories, out of fat. Eliminate 250 fat calories. Add enough exercise to burn 250 calories a day. That's a net withdrawal from your fat bank of 500 calories a day.

2. If you are considerably overweight, eliminate 500 food calories and exercise off 500 calories each day for a net withdrawal of 1,000 calories a day. You need to work out with this, though under a doctor's supervision. Your diet should also have some medical monitoring.

3. A pound of fat equals 3,500 calories. In scenario number one, you create a deficit of 3,500 calories per week. Theoretically, you burn off a pound of fat each

week, or 52 pounds a year. However, while this sounds great in theory, it *does not* work this way in actuality. In fact, this *will* happen for the first few weeks, but you quickly adjust and your metabolism slows down to save body fat. If you don't weight train, your body may burn muscle *instead of* fat!

4. In scenario number two, you create a two-pound-per-week deficit. Don't try to lose more than two pounds per week.

5. Many doctors say that you shouldn't eat too much protein or carbs or they will be stored as fat. However, as mentioned, it's difficult *if almost impossible to store either excess protein or unrefined carbohydrates as fat! I used the fruit example earlier. And as for too much protein—I know of no obese person who got that way because all they ate were 10 cans of water-packed tuna each day.*

Ten cans of tuna provide over 400 grams of protein per day, by far an excess for anyone, yet you would not get fat from this, if it's all you ate. You might get sick, but you would not get fat. You also would hate tuna forever!

If you ate 20 servings of high-quality protein powder with water every day (400 grams of protein), you wouldn't get fat either! It would be a waste of money and time, though, and you'd visit the bathroom a lot. Everything is taken out of context. Too much protein doesn't mean much in weight control if you don't eat enough calories. Four hundred grams of protein yields about 1,600 calories of energy. How-

Low-fat or nonfat commercial cooking sprays are a great innovation.

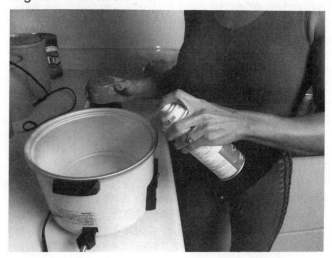

ever, 400 grams of fat yields over 3,600 calories.

In an average daily diet, if you eat 100 grams of protein, 300 grams of carbs and 150 fat grams, you get about 3,000 calories a day. Of those 3,000 calories, only a limited number should be in the form of fat or simple sugars.

On the protein issue, I would be remiss if I didn't talk about possible medical concerns some doctors have with liver and kidney function. For sure, most people probably consume more protein than they need and if you have a high-protein diet, you do need to drink more water and perhaps take a calcium supplement. Most doctors maintain that if your kidneys are healthy, excess protein is excreted, not easily converted into fat and stored.

Consider fruits and vegetables. You could eat 30 oranges or apples a day (3,000 calories) and *not* get fat. However, if you ate 3,000 calories of Hershey's chocolate bars, you'd likely gain fat because simple sugars cause your pancreas to produce insulin and insulin tends to promote body fat (not to mention all the fat in those candy bars)!

Simple sugars, like candy bars, are almost *always* associated with fat calories. High-protein foods may put weight on you because they are also associated with fat, as for example red meats.

6. If you are active, simple sugars are metabolized for energy. To have your cake and eat it too, work out! As I've mentioned already, carbohydrates and protein yield about four calories of energy per gram when they are oxidized for energy. Fat yields more than *nine* calories per gram.

7. A balanced diet with a variety of foods provides energy and satiety, as well as nutrients. Food supplement vitamins and minerals *do not* provide energy because they're noncaloric. They don't satiate you either! However, in certain situations supplements are necessary.

Supplements might be used when you are ill or recovering from an extended illness; when you are under severe emotional, mental or physical stress; during pregnancy; under very heavy work loads where you sweat profusely and on diets where your nutrient levels are down.

8. Eat like a king in the morning, a queen in the afternoon and a poor man at night! Exercise like a poor man working his fields in the morning, carry on like a queen during the day and relax like a king at night! Don't skip meals *or* workouts.

9. Some unfortunate individuals with slow biological set points (doctors believe each of us has a built-in set point in our hypothalamus that governs appetite, metabolic rate, satiety and body weight) need special medical counseling. Some of these individuals also have hormonal problems or enzymatic discrepancies at their muscle cell level, which makes them gain fat *in spite* of low-calorie diets. However, these individuals *will* benefit from good nutrition and exercise, in addition to medications.

If you fall into this category, you *must* work with your physician. Don't be discouraged! You can do it.

HOW MANY CALORIES? HOW MANY GRAMS OF FAT, PROTEIN AND CARBOHYDRATES? THE RULE OF 10.

You can estimate how many calories you need and a lot of doctors and nutritionists have formulas for this, but they don't mean much. Energy requirements for two individuals who weigh the same can actually vary by 100 percent!

A 200-pound man might need 2,000 calories a day to meet his energy requirements. Another 200-pound man may need

Add some fruit to this plate and you have a perfect meal—high in carbs, vitamins and minerals, low in fat and moderate in protein.

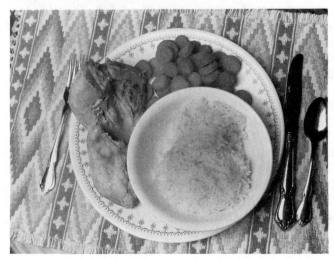

4,000 calories. To estimate your BMR (basal metabolic rate—the daily calories you burn at rest), multiply your weight by 10. The BMR is where you get tremendous deviation between two individuals, but the rule of 10 is a fair estimate.

If you have a desk job and an inactive lifestyle, add another 25 percent to your BMR. If you are moderately active, add 50 percent (or multiply your weight by 15). If you are very active, as for example a laborer, or you train regularly and hard, multiply your weight by 20.

A 130-pound woman who weight trains and teaches three classes of aerobics every other day needs at least 2,500–3,000 calories a day. When I was competing for Ms. Olympia, I could eat over 4,000 calories a day and still *lose* weight!

For athletes, as I mentioned much earlier, eat between 1–1.5 grams of protein per kilogram of body weight each day. No more than 20 percent of your total calories should come from fat. So, if you need 1,500 calories a day, take 20 percent of that, which is 300 calories. Fat provides nine calories per gram. Divide nine into 300. This is about 33 grams of fat per day. As far as grams of carbohydrates go, if you are active you can eat as many carbohydrates as you want, as long as they're not simple sugars like candies, cookies, pies, etc.

Unless your doctor declares a medical emergency, never eat less than 1,000 calories a day. Unless you are very knowledgeable about combining calorie-dense foods, a diet this low in calories will probably not provide the carbs, fats, proteins, fiber, vitamins and minerals you need for daily maintenance and health. Besides which, as I mentioned earlier, you'll lose valuable muscle on such a low-calorie diet.

POPULAR COMMERCIAL DIET PROGRAMS

1. Jenny Craig

Jenny Craig pre-prepared frozen meals (together with snacks) provide 900–1,200 calories. There is no specific time that you are required to follow the diet. Jenny Craig does require a couple of visits each week to pick up the planned meals and to be educated on exercise and food preparation.

2. Nutri/System

Nutri/System meals come in small pouches and are usually freeze-dried. There's roughly 1,000–1,200 calories provided in one day. You can stay with the program as long as you like. Clients are required to attend weekly sessions on food preparation and behavior.

3. Weight Watchers

Weight Watchers is based on regular food. Total daily calories average 1,000–1,350. However, the client is able to use food provided by Weight Watchers, at their option. Organized meetings last over a 10-week period, once a week. Education focuses on behavior adjustments, exercise and food preparation.

4. Medifast

Medifast provides a low 450-calorie liquid diet with an additional optional caloric supplement of 850 calories. The program lasts 16 weeks. Because of the low-calorie program, all clients must undergo physician tests consisting of electrocardiogram, urinalysis and blood tests. Clients participate in one-hour classes each week on exercise and food behavior modification.

5. Optifast

This plan provides between 420 and 800 calories a day, depending on the servings. The program lasts one year with some periods devoted to just the supplement and some time with normal food.

In my opinion, these disciplined, organized diet centers and plans are very helpful. For many, though, they aren't practical and there's a lot of recidivism when the program ends. Adopt a new "lifestyle" in which exercise and eating fit into your values, energy and time frame, with your specific goal. You have a better shot at long-term weight control and health if you learn about food values and how to put nutritional foods together. It's also important to know why you shouldn't eat certain foods—what foods are high calorie or have hidden fats, sugars and sodium.

Low-calorie diets always fail! It's better to eat the right foods, and still be able to eat a lot of calories, as long as they're low-fat foods included with exercise.

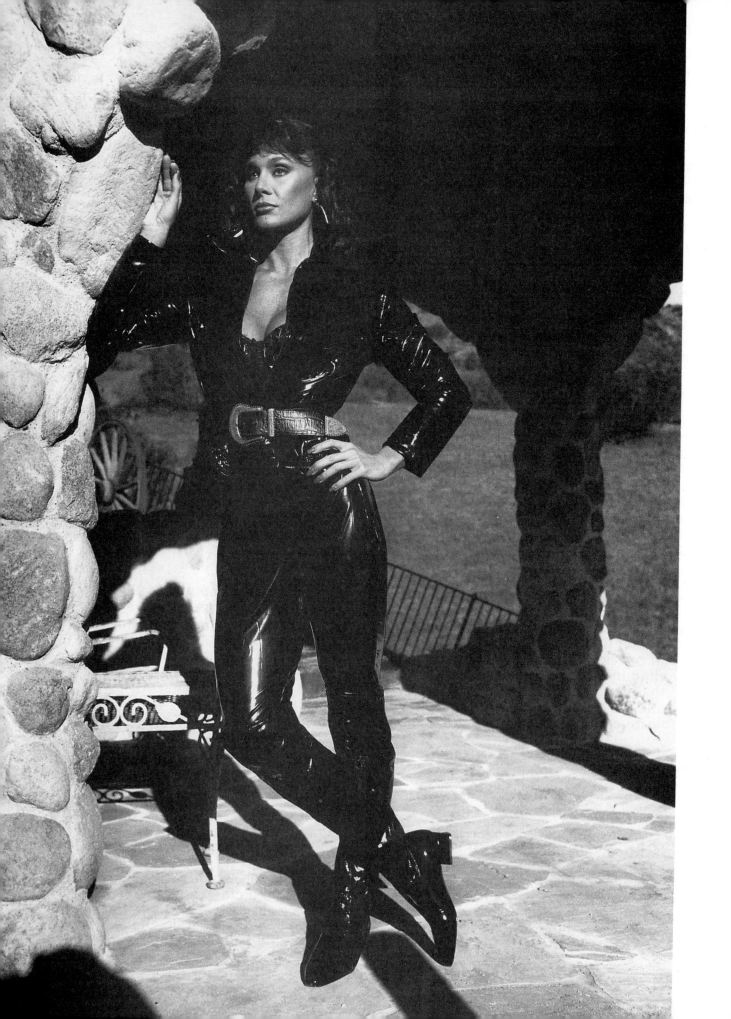

10
NUTRITION: YOUR FINAL STEP

Eating right can be confusing. However, if you really want healthy nutrition in your life, you have to learn what is in food, which foods are high in fat, calories and sodium, etc. You also need to know how to construct food plans that meet all your daily needs. With all of that in mind, let's get down to business.

THE GOOD, BAD AND UGLY: THE FOODS WE EAT

Product	Fat (grams)	Calories	Sodium (milligrams)
French Fries (3 oz)	2–17	90–300	15–500

We might as well start with one of our most popular fast foods. According to the Tuft's University Diet & Nutrition Healthletter, there's a big difference in various french-fry brands.

Three ounces of Ore-Ida Lite french fries have just 90 calories, two grams of fat and 30 grams of sodium. Another brand of Ore-Ida actually has less sodium in three ounces, but more calories and slightly more fat. McDonald's fries contain 320 calories in three and a half ounces with 17 grams of fat. Four ounces of Burger King fries have 340 calories and 20 grams of fat. Ore-Ida Crispers contain 535 milligrams of sodium in just three ounces. Ouch! Out of the 17 grams of fat in the McDonald's fries, four grams are saturated, but there is zero cholesterol. On a percentage basis, 48 percent of the food is fat! So, if you must eat french fries, get the light variety!

For comparison, Wendy's plain baked potato contains about 250 calories with 60 milligrams of sodium and *zero* grams of fat. However, if you add butter and salt, forget it. Let's continue with some fast foods.

Fast Foods

Product	Fat (grams)	Calories	Sodium (milligrams)
Arby's Chicken Breast Sandwich	25	493	1019

A pensive Ms. Olympia in her backyard gazebo.

175

Product	Fat (grams)	Calories	Sodium (milligrams)
Burger King Chicken Tenders (6 pieces)	10	204	—
Burger King Croissant-wich with Sausage	40	538	1042
Burger King Whopper with Cheese	43	711	—
Carl's Jr. BBQ Chicken Sandwich	4–5	320	955
Hardee's Bacon Cheese-burger	33	556	—
Hardee's Big Country Breakfast Sausage	72	1005	1950
Hardee's Chicken Stix (6 pieces)	10	234	—
Hardee's Grilled Chicken Sandwich	12	330	1240
Jack in the Box Grilled Chicken Fillet Sandwich	16	408	1130
Jack in the Box Ultimate Cheese-burger	69	942	1176
McDonald's Biscuit with Sausage & Egg	36	529	1250
McDonald's Chef Salad	12	231	490
McDonald's Hamburger	10	260	460
McDonald's Hot Cakes with Butter/Syrup	8	413	640
McDonald's McChicken Sandwich	26	490	780
McDonald's Mc DLT	42	674	1170
McDonald's Quarter Pounder with Cheese	30	520	1150
Roy Rogers Bar Burger	39	611	—
Roy Rogers Roast Beef Sandwich	10	317	—
Taco Bell Bean Burrito with Green Sauce	10	351	763
Taco Bell Chicken Fajita	10	226	703
Taco Bell Steak Fajita	11	234	485
Taco Bell Taco	10	183	276
Taco Bell Taco Light	28	410	594
Taco Bell Taco Salad without Shell	30	520	1431
Taco Bell Taco Salad with Shell	61	941	1662
Wendy's Bacon Swiss Burger	44	710	—
Wendy's Big Classic with Cheese	40	640	1310
Wendy's Chicken Breast Sandwich	18	430	705

Product	Fat (grams)	Calories	Sodium (milligrams)
Wendy's Plain Single	16	350	—
Wendy's Triple Cheeseburger	70	1040	1848

Most doctors recommend a daily sodium intake of about 2,400 milligrams. Most of you consume far too much sodium. Excess sodium may be a factor for some people in developing high blood pressure or adversely affecting high-blood-pressure control.

If you are supposed to eat only 20 percent of your total calories as fat, where do you sit eating fast foods? Well, you sit on your fatty acids!

Consider a 160-pound average man. He needs between 1,600 and 2,400 calories each day. Let's figure 2,000 calories. Twenty percent of 2,000 is 400 calories. Fat yields more than nine calories per gram. Four hundred divided by nine (9.2 actually) is about 44 grams. That's your daily maximum for fat. You could have one Wendy's Big Classic with Cheese and nothing else for the day. If you had a Wendy's Triple Cheeseburger on Monday, in terms of fat, you couldn't eat anything again until Wednesday! And that's allowing 20 percent fat—many experts say 10 percent fat is enough.

THE BAD NEWS CONTINUES

Here's another list to depress you:

Margarine

Product	Calories	Total Fat (grams)	Saturated Fat (grams)
Tub (1 Tbsp):			
Blue Bonnet Spread	80	8	2
Country Morning Blend	90	10	3
Diet Fleischmann's	50	6	1
Imperial Light Spread	60	6	2
Parkay Spread	60	7	1
Promise	90	10	1
Promise Extra Light	50	6	1
Shedd's Country Crock	70	7	1
Whipped Blue Bonnet Spread	50	6	1
Stick (1 Tbsp):			
Country Morning Blend	100	11	3
Promise Extra Light	50	6	1
Whipped Blue Bonnet	70	7	2

Butter has 100 calories per tablespoon with 11 grams of fat, of which seven are saturated. Butter-Buds and Molly McButter have 21–24 calories per tablespoon with *no* fat at all! You shouldn't have more than 30–40 grams of fat a day and no more than 20 grams of saturated fat. If one pat of butter has seven grams of saturated fat, how much do you eat each day just from butter? If you spread a bit on your morning toast and some on your evening potato, you're already saturated.

Margarines are higher in polyunsaturated fats than butter. There's some evidence that polyunsaturated fats lower cholesterol. My opinion is that you shouldn't use any butter or margarine, or very little. Bread is fine without butter. So are potatoes. If somehow everyone could stop eating butter, fat consumption would go way down.

And, don't destroy a good treat like popcorn by adding butter and salt.

Microwave Popcorn (one cup, popped)

Product	Calories	% Calories from Fat	Sodium (milligrams)
Jolly time Natural	53	56	60
Newman's Own Natural	45	48	0
Orville Redenbacher's Natural	33	53	97
Planters Natural	47	61	187
Pop Secret Light Natural	23	39	38
Weight Watchers	25	9	1

How much difference is there between air and oil-popped popcorn? According to *Men's Fitness* magazine, four cups of plain, air-popped corn has 109 calories without any fat and 5.2 grams of fiber. Four cups of plain oil-popped corn contain 132 calories with 5.6 grams of fat and 4.4 grams of fiber. Who eats just four cups of popcorn? When I snack on popcorn, I probably eat at least 10 cups, maybe 15. What about you?

For comparison: 10 potato chips have 162 calories and 11.3 grams of fat!! When you sit down to munch on chips, it's easy to eat half a bag if you don't watch it. The fat just piles up. Potato chips and french fries are the worst—the toilet bowl of foods.

It gets worse. Let's look at those terrible candies.

Junk Food Sweets (ounces)

Product	Calories	% Calories from Fat
Almond Joy (1.8)	250	47
Baby Ruth (2.2)	300	39
Fi-Bar (1)	100	28
Hershey's Chocolate Bar (1.7)	250	50
Hershey's Kisses (5)	122	28
Kraft Caramel (3)	105	26

Product	Calories	% Calories from Fat
Mars (1.8)	200	42
Milk Duds (10)	129	31
Milky Way (2)	280	35
M&M's Peanut (12)	141	47
M&M's Plain (33)	146	43
Mr. Goodbar (1.9)	300	60
Nestlé Bit-o-Honey (1.7)	200	18
Nestlé Crunch (1.4)	210	43
Peanut Butter Snickers (1.8)	280	58
Snickers (2.1)	280	45
Sugar Babies (20)	113	10
Sweetarts (33)	120	0
3 Musketeers (2.1)	260	28

Unfortunately, our taste buds are our worst enemy. Almost all candy is too high in simple sugar and fats, a deadly combination. While I know this is true, I can't resist a Snickers myself now and then. Like I said earlier though, if you want your cake and to eat it too, you have to work out hard and regularly.

Some Common Salad Dressings (one tablespoon)

Product	Calories	Fat (grams)	Cholesterol (milligrams)	Sodium (milligrams)
Chunky Blue Cheese (Kraft)	60	6	5	230
Chunky French (Kraft)	60	5–6	0	115

Product	Calories	Fat (grams)	Cholesterol (milligrams)	Sodium (milligrams)
Regular Italian (Kraft)	70	7–8	0	300
Regular Ranch (Kraft)	80	7–10	7.5	133
Thousand Island (Kraft)	70	4–5	5	140

Do you use one tablespoon of salad dressing at the salad bar? I bet not. Most people probably use close to 8–10 tablespoons. You could get up to 70–80 grams of fat just from the salad dressing at the salad bar! Bring your own diet dressing. Most of the reduced-calorie dressings have less than one gram of fat per tablespoon. Over a long time, it makes a big difference.

More Common Food Values

Food	Calories	Carbohydrates	Fat (grams)	Protein
Lean Beef (4 oz)	260	0	20	20
Cheese (4 oz)	455	20	40	10
Chicken (4 oz)	200	0	14	23
Cottage Cheese (8 oz)	220	4–5	1–3	42
Egg	80	0	6	6
Fish (4 oz)	84	0	0	20
Ham (4 oz)	380	0	30	20
Hamburger (4 oz)	260	0	20	19
Ice Cream (8 oz)	360	35	22	5
Liver (4 oz)	240	11	9	27
Lobster (4 oz)	100	0	2	20
Peanuts (8 oz)	820	32	60	40

Food	Calories	Carbohydrates	Fat (grams)	Protein
Pork (4 oz)	325	0	25	25
Regular Milk (8 oz)	165	12	10	8
Turkey (4 oz)	280	0	20	24
Veal (4 oz)	210	0	12	25

TOO MUCH JAVA?

As if fats and simple sugars aren't bad enough, too much caffeine in your food and beverages can alter your blood sugar, cause nervousness, change your appetite, cause headaches (especially when you try to stop), aggravate and perhaps cause cystic breast disease, raise your blood pressure and, some scientists feel, put you at heightened risk for heart attacks, although the jury is still out on this.

Caffeine Content in Popular Beverages/Medications (in milligrams)

Coca-Cola (12 oz)	45
Decaffeinated Coffee (5 oz)	3–6
Drip Coffee (5 oz)	120–150
Excedrin Tablet	130
Instant Coffee (5 oz)	50–100
Instant Tea (5 oz)	15–30
Jolt (12 oz)	72
Mountain Dew (12 oz)	55
No-Doz Tablet	100
Pepsi-Cola (12 oz)	38
Percolated Coffee (5 oz)	70–125
RC Cola (12 oz)	35
Sugar-free Dr Pepper	40
Vivarin Tablet	200

Calories in Popular Beverages

Diet Coke (12 oz)	1
Gatorade (8 oz)	40
Hi-C (6 oz)	90
Kool Aid (8 oz)	70
Lemonade (8 oz)	100
Mineral Water (12 oz)	0
Unsweetened Tea (8 oz)	3

HOW TO PUT YOUR PERSONAL NUTRITION PLAN TOGETHER!

Define your goals. If your goal is to lose fat weight, work out with aerobics and weights and follow a nutrition plan that meets your caloric needs (use the rule of 10, according to your body weight and then add calories according to your activity; subtract calories according to the rate you wish to lose or better yet, visit a physiologist and have your BMR determined). Your nutrition plan must also include enough protein, carbohydrates, fats, vitamins, minerals and water.

Case One: A sample 1,200-calorie/day food plan.

Breakfast:

- Sliced fruit with medium-size bowl of oatmeal. Use skim milk, sugar substitute.
- One poached egg, three times a week only.
- One cup decaffeinated coffee or tea.
- One large glass of water.
- One multiple-vitamin/mineral supplement.
- Small protein drink with fresh orange juice.

Lunch:

- Open-face tuna or turkey sandwich on whole-wheat or rye bread. A small amount of margarine is allowed, but no mayo!
- Two large glasses of water.
- One cup coffee or tea.
- Medium-size dinner salad with low-calorie dressing. Include cucumbers, carrots, celery, lentils, onions and tomatoes.

Dinner:

- Medium chicken breast (remove the skin) or four ounces of baked fish or lean hamburger.
- Baked potato with a couple dabs of low-fat cottage cheese, chives and pepper.
- Medium-size bowl of vegetables (no butter).
- Mineral water.

Case Two: A sample 1,200-calorie/day food plan.

This plan provides 150 grams of carbohydrates, 65 grams of protein and 40 grams of fat. Remember your math: When the carbs are burned: 150 grams × 4 calories per gram (600 calories); plus when the protein is burned: 65 grams × 4 calories per gram (260 calories) and when the fat is burned: 40 grams × 9 calories per gram (360 calories).

Breakfast:

- One cup orange juice.
- 1 or 2 slices of whole-wheat or rye toast, light margarine.
- One cup skim milk with protein powder supplement.
- One multiple-vitamin supplement.

Lunch:

- One pear.
- One cup of skim milk.
- One-ounce slice of cheese.
- One cup of carrots.
- One dinner salad with diet dressing.
- One serving of yellow vegetables.

Dinner:

- Baked chicken without skin.
- Baked potato
- One cup broccoli or asparagus.
- One peach, apple or banana.
- Mineral water with lemon twist.

Case Three: A sample 1,500-calorie/day food plan.

This plan provides approximately 165 grams of carbohydrates, 90 grams of protein, 40—50 grams of fat.

Breakfast:

- Half cup of orange juice.

- Small banana.
- Two slices of rye toast with pat of diet margarine.
- Small bowl of high-fiber cereal.
- One cup skim milk.
- Half cup low-fat cottage cheese.

Lunch:

- Turkey sandwich on rye.
- Large bowl of mixed vegetables, including corn and peas.
- Apple or orange.
- Cup of skim milk.

Dinner:

- Chicken breast (approximately four ounces).
- Mashed potatoes without butter (white gravy allowed).
- Cup of broccoli, brussels sprouts, cauliflower or asparagus.
- Large salad.
- Four ounces of white wine or mineral water.

Snack:

- Any fruit or air-popped light popcorn.

Case Four: A sample 1,500-calorie/day food plan.

Breakfast:

- Two slices of whole-wheat toast; half a melon or grapefruit; six ounces of fresh juice.
- Cup of skim milk with one ounce of protein supplement.

Lunch:

- Turkey- or chicken-salad sandwich with low-calorie condiment.
- Nonfat yogurt.
- Half a melon.
- Cup of skim milk.

Dinner:

- Salad with vinegar dressing.
- Baked potato.
- Small, lean steak, all fat removed.
- Small serving of vegetables.
- Mineral water or grapefruit juice.

Snack:

- Half cup of frozen-yogurt dessert or two cups of air-popped light popcorn.

Case Five: A sample 1,500-calorie/day food plan.

Breakfast:

- Two cups strawberries.
- One slice whole-wheat toast.
- Cup of skim milk.

Lunch:

- Cup of vegetable soup.
- Apple.
- Plate of pasta with side of low-fat cottage cheese.
- Cup of skim milk.
- Small salad.

Dinner:

- Skinless chicken breast, 4–6 ounces baked fish or 4–6 ounces broiled steak (fat removed and meat squeezed of excess oil).
- Large bowl of vegetables.
- Cup of skim milk.

Case Six: A sample 1,800-calorie/day food plan.

Breakfast:
- Bowl of bran flakes with low-fat milk.
- Two pieces of whole-wheat toast.
- One whole egg or three egg whites with no yolks.

Lunch:
- Bowl of rice.
- Large salad.
- Large protein drink with skim milk.
- Banana.

Dinner:
- Two pieces of baked chicken without skin.
- Two cups of fresh vegetables including mushrooms, onions, celery, squash, green peppers, carrots and bean sprouts.
- Baked potato.
- Small glass of white wine.

Snack:
- Air popcorn, fruit or rice cakes.

Case Seven: A sample 2,000-calorie/day food plan.

Breakfast:
- Orange or banana.
- Omelette with mushrooms, onions, diced ham, 2–3 egg whites, but only one yolk.
- Two slices of whole-wheat toast with pat of margarine.
- Cup of skim milk with protein powder.

Lunch:
- Tuna-salad sandwich.
- Large mixed salad.
- Apple.
- Juice or mineral water.

Dinner:
- Four-ounce broiled steak.
- Large baked potato.
- Large plate of steamed vegetables.
- Glass of 2-percent milk.

Snack:
- Fruit, yogurt, popcorn or skim-milk protein drink.

WHAT ABOUT THE SODIUM THING?

On a daily basis, 2,400–2,500 milligrams of sodium is the upper limit approved by most doctors. Let's look at some sodium examples.

Here is the sodium content of a typical American breakfast (in milligrams):

1. Two fried eggs	350
2. 2 or 3 strips of bacon	350
3. English muffin/butter	320
4. Glass of orange juice	Trace
5. Coffee	Trace
Total sodium	920 mg.

Here is the sodium content of a typical American lunch or dinner (in milligrams):

1. Serving of chips or french fries with catsup	850
2. Cheeseburger with condiments	1200
3. Commercial-size pickle	900
4. Flavored milk shake or malted milk	550
Total sodium	3500 mg.

Here is a low-sodium breakfast:

1. Bowl of shredded wheat with skim milk.
2. Any grouping of fruit, melon, nectarines, strawberries, peach and/or oranges.
3. Juice.
4. Coffee.

This meal provides less than 500 milligrams of sodium.

Here is an example of a low-sodium lunch or dinner:

1. Serving of broccoli.
2. Large salad with diet dressing.
3. Bowl of steamed rice.
4. Glass of white wine.
5. Fruit plate.
6. Protein supplement with fruit juice.

To keep your sodium down, avoid these foods: ham, bacon, smoked meats like bologna, butter, catsup, most cold sugared cereals, cheeses, fried meats, potato chips, french fries, corned beef hash, hash browns, crackers, doughnuts, ground beef, hot dogs, pickles, pork, salamis, creamy soups, ribs, steaks and ice creams and other desserts.

FINALLY: LET'S MAKE EATING PRACTICAL!

There are practical ways to cut fat in the way you eat. As a concluding note, if you follow these simple tips, you'll do yourself a *big* favor health-wise, the way you look and feel!

1. **Don't ever use regular mayonnaise again.** One tablespoon of mayo saturates you with over 10 grams of fat and 100 calories. Since the taste is the same, use light mayo. Most of these brands provide half as much fat and calories or less! Use low-calorie mayo in all your cooking when mayo is called for.

2. **Don't fry your foods; boil or bake.** Sauté or steam your vegetables.

3. **Don't salt vegetables, meat or soups,** even if recipes call for it.

4. **Cut all visible fat off your meat before cooking.**

5. **When you order meat, before eating it, wrap it in napkins and squeeze out excess oil.** Do the same with hamburger buns.

6. **Skip french fries and potato chips as long as the sun continues to shine.**

7. **If you crave doughnuts or chocolate candy bars, decide to eat no more than one each per week.**

8. **Don't add butter or margarine to your hot baked potato.** Let your food cool first— you'll use less butter. Try to eliminate extra butter on any and all foods.

9. **Don't add gravy to your meat or potatoes.**

10. **When making casseroles, don't use creamy, thick, salty soups.** Make your own sauces for casseroles with skim milk, vegetables, flour and chicken or turkey bits.

11. **Substitute de-skinned chicken and turkey bits for red meats in recipes.**

12. **Use low-calorie salad dressings at all times.**

13. **Eat more baked fish (without tartar sauce).**

14. **Eat steamed vegetables and fresh fruit to your heart's content.** Doing so will make your heart content!

15. **Eat protein from low-fat sources (egg whites, beans, legumes, skim milk, tuna, lentils, corn, de-skinned chicken and turkey, fish and even commercial protein powders.**

16. **Skim milk has less than a gram of fat and 90 calories per eight ounces.** Whole milk has 150 calories and eight fat grams. *Utterly* ridiculous! Get the picture?

17. **Read and study everything in my book again!** Good luck to all of you.

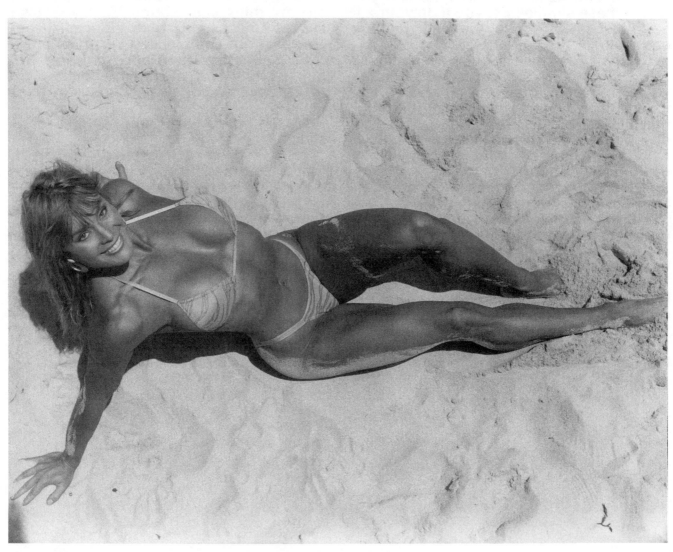

Cory exudes California health and has some fun in the white sand and sun.

Index

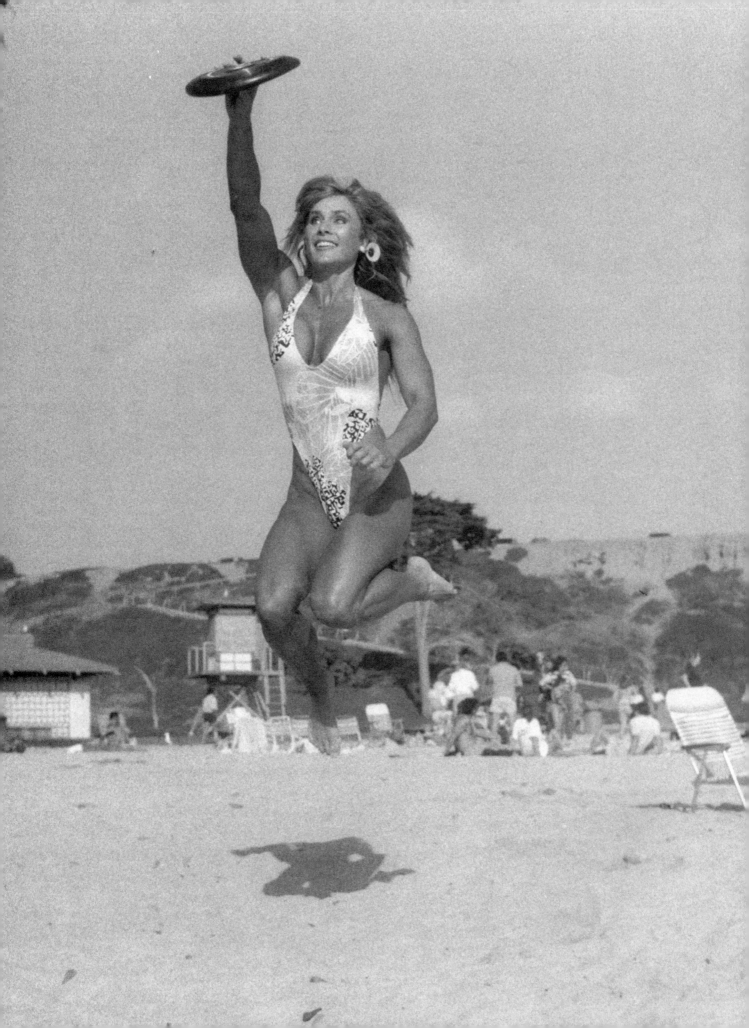

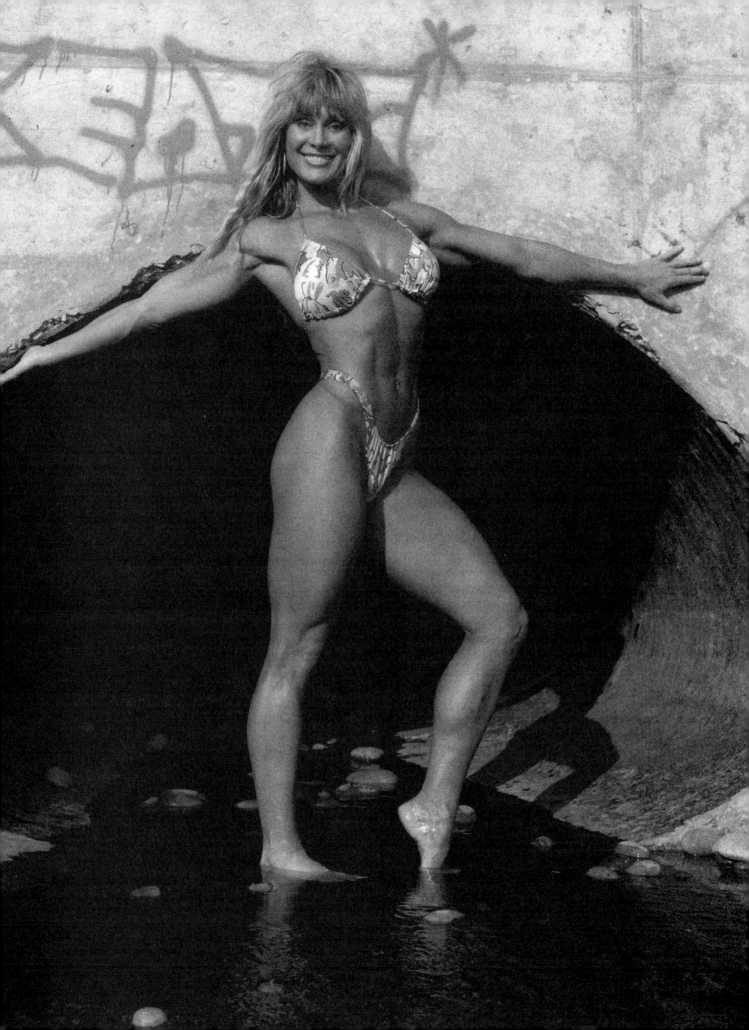

OTHER BOOKS OF INTEREST

CORY EVERSON'S FAT-FREE AND FIT

by Cory Everson with Carole Jacobs 0-399-51858-4/$15.00

Cory Everson, internationally acclaimed fitness expert and six-time Ms. Olympia, shares her secrets to a fabulous, fat-free and fit body.

CORY EVERSON'S WORKOUT

by Corinna Everson and Jeff Everson, Ph.D. 0-399-51684-0/$16.95

An innovative fitness program from six-time Ms. Olympia and television star Cory Everson. More than 150 black-and-white photographs.

A WOMAN'S BOOK OF STRENGTH

by Karen Andes 0-399-51899-1/$14.00

"Karen Andes is a rare combination of expertise and sensitivity....This should have been the first fitness book ever done." —Cher

A unique, empowering guide that shows women how to mine the powers of the heart, mind, spirit, and body.

A WOMAN'S BOOK OF POWER

by Karen Andes   0-399-52372-3/$14.00

A step-by-step guide that explores the round, soft movements that feel more natural to the female body. Incorporates Middle Eastern dance, other ancient sacred dances, as well as martial arts and yoga.

CALLANETICS FIT FOREVER

by Callan Pinckney 0-399-52263-8/$13.00

Introducing Cardio-Callanetics, a low-impact aerobic exercise to benefit the cardio-vascular system. Revolutionizing the way women will exercise for the rest of their lives.

SIX WEEK FAT-TO-MUSCLE MAKEOVER

by Ellington Darden, Ph.d. 0-399-51562-3/$11.95

A safe and healthful diet-and-exercise plan that actually changes the body's fat-to-muscle ratio. Includes menu plans, recipes, exercise routines, and inspiring before-and-after photos.

TO ORDER CALL: 1-800-788-6262, ext. 1. Refer to Ad #603

Perigee Books
A member of Penguin Putnam Inc.
200 Madison Avenue
New York, NY 10016

*Prices subject to change